NEUROSCIENCE RESEARCH PROGRESS

TUMORS OF THE CENTRAL NERVOUS SYSTEM

CLINICAL ASPECTS AND SYMPTOM MANAGEMENT

NEUROSCIENCE RESEARCH PROGRESS

Additional books and e-books in this series can be found
on Nova's website under the Series tab.

NEUROSCIENCE RESEARCH PROGRESS

TUMORS OF THE CENTRAL NERVOUS SYSTEM

CLINICAL ASPECTS AND SYMPTOM MANAGEMENT

JAMES A. REED
EDITOR

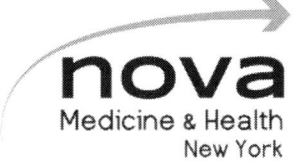

Copyright © 2021 by Nova Science Publishers, Inc.

All rights reserved. No part of this book may be reproduced, stored in a retrieval system or transmitted in any form or by any means: electronic, electrostatic, magnetic, tape, mechanical photocopying, recording or otherwise without the written permission of the Publisher.

We have partnered with Copyright Clearance Center to make it easy for you to obtain permissions to reuse content from this publication. Simply navigate to this publication's page on Nova's website and locate the "Get Permission" button below the title description. This button is linked directly to the title's permission page on copyright.com. Alternatively, you can visit copyright.com and search by title, ISBN, or ISSN.

For further questions about using the service on copyright.com, please contact:
Copyright Clearance Center
Phone: +1-(978) 750-8400   Fax: +1-(978) 750-4470   E-mail: info@copyright.com.

NOTICE TO THE READER

The Publisher has taken reasonable care in the preparation of this book, but makes no expressed or implied warranty of any kind and assumes no responsibility for any errors or omissions. No liability is assumed for incidental or consequential damages in connection with or arising out of information contained in this book. The Publisher shall not be liable for any special, consequential, or exemplary damages resulting, in whole or in part, from the readers' use of, or reliance upon, this material. Any parts of this book based on government reports are so indicated and copyright is claimed for those parts to the extent applicable to compilations of such works.

Independent verification should be sought for any data, advice or recommendations contained in this book. In addition, no responsibility is assumed by the Publisher for any injury and/or damage to persons or property arising from any methods, products, instructions, ideas or otherwise contained in this publication.

This publication is designed to provide accurate and authoritative information with regard to the subject matter covered herein. It is sold with the clear understanding that the Publisher is not engaged in rendering legal or any other professional services. If legal or any other expert assistance is required, the services of a competent person should be sought. FROM A DECLARATION OF PARTICIPANTS JOINTLY ADOPTED BY A COMMITTEE OF THE AMERICAN BAR ASSOCIATION AND A COMMITTEE OF PUBLISHERS.

Additional color graphics may be available in the e-book version of this book.

Library of Congress Cataloging-in-Publication Data

ISBN: 978-1-53619-628-3

Published by Nova Science Publishers, Inc. † New York

CONTENTS

Preface vii

Chapter 1 Embryonal Tumor with Multilayered Rosettes, C19MC-Altered 1
Emad Ababneh and Richard Prayson

Chapter 2 Dysembryoplastic Neuroepithelial Tumor (DNET): A Clinicopathologic Review 17
Mrinal M. Sarwate and Richard A. Prayson

Chapter 3 Rosai-Dorfman Disease of the Central Nervous System 31
Ahmed Bakhshwin and Richard A. Prayson

Chapter 4 The Clinical and Pathologic Features of Angiocentric Glioma 45
Richard Prayson

Chapter 5 Chordoid Gliomas: Pathological and Clinical Aspects 57
Anas M. Saad and Richard A. Prayson

Chapter 6	Dysplastic Gangliocytoma of the Cerebellum (Lhermitte-Duclos Disease): A Clinicopathologic Review *Richard A. Prayson*	**69**
Chapter 7	Clinicopathologic Review of Cerebellar Liponeurocytoma *Richard A. Prayson*	**81**
Index		**95**

Preface

This book contains seven chapters, each of which provides information about tumors of the central nervous system. Chapter One reviews the clinical, pathological, molecular and prognostic features of Embryonal Tumor with Multilayered Rosettes (EMTR), an aggressive, WHO grade IV tumor. Chapter Two reviews the clinicopathologic features and differential diagnoses of Dysembryoplastic neuroepithelial tumor (DNET), a rare low grade glioneuronal neoplasm which mostly affects the temporal lobe. Chapter Three reviews the clinical and pathologic features of Rosai-Dorfman disease (RDD), a rare, benign, idiopathic lymphohistiocytic proliferative disease. Chapter Four reviews the clinical and pathologic features of the rare central nervous system neoplasm called angiocentric gliomas. Chapter Five reviews the histological and clinical features of chordoid gliomas, which are rare neoplasms of the central nervous system. Chapter Six provides a clinicopathologic review of dysplastic cerebellar gangliocytomas, also known as Lhermitte-Duclos disease. Finally, Chapter Seven reviews the clinicopathologic features of cerebellar liponeurocytoma, a rare cerebellar tumor which is marked by admixed neurocytic and lipoma-like components.

Chapter 1 - Embryonal Tumor with Multilayered Rosettes (EMTR) is an aggressive, WHO grade IV tumor. It was defined as a distinct entity in the most recent WHO classification of tumors of the brain and spinal cord in 2016. Previously, it was diagnosed under the umbrella of the primitive neuroectodermal tumors (PNET) family with heterogeneous morphological patterns of medulloepithelioma, ependymoblastoma, and embryonal tumor with abundant neuropil and true rosettes. The growing evidence that this group of tumors shares the characteristic chromosome 19 miRNA cluster (*C19MC*) amplification as well as their distinct clinical behavior made the creation of this entity possible. The diagnosis of this entity is still challenging to make, whether for its rarity or the overlapping histology and clinical features with other embryonal tumors. Furthermore, the ongoing discovery of further genetic driving events, for instance, *DICER1* mutations, may lead to refinements in the prognosis and potential therapy. In this chapter, the authors are going to discuss this entity in detail, reviewing the clinical, pathological, molecular and prognostic features of this rare entity.

Chapter 2 - Dysembryoplastic neuroepithelial tumor (DNET) is a rare low grade (World Health Organization grade I) glioneuronal neoplasm which mostly affects the temporal lobe. It usually presents in the 2nd or 3rd decades of life and is slightly more common in males. Patients with DNET typically present with focal seizures which may be pharmacoresistant and may warrant surgical excision. On imaging studies, DNET appears to be confined to the cerebral cortex. There may be thickening of the cortex with well demarcated nodules, some showing internal nodularity with a pseudocystic, bubbly appearance due to the mucoid material. Histopathologically, the tumor is composed of oligodendroglial-like cells, patterned intracortical nodules and "floating neurons" seen in the mucoid material. DNET is subdivided into simple and complex variants. The simple variant is composed of specific glioneuronal element only, while the complex variant has glial nodules in addition to specific glioneuronal elements. Coexistent focal cortical dysplasia is a common finding in the adjacent brain tissue. Differential diagnoses of DNET include oligodendroglioma and ganglioglioma. This chapter will review the clinicopathologic features and differential diagnoses of DNET.

Chapter 3 - Rosai-Dorfman disease (RDD) is a rare, benign, idiopathic lymphohistiocytic proliferative disease that has been reported to involve virtually all anatomic sites including, although seldom, the central nervous system. It tends to present as a solitary mass or as multiple dural masses with a predilection for the cerebral convexities, cavernous sinuses, as well as parasagittal, sellar and suprasellar regions. It is therefore very understandable that these lesions are often thought to be meningiomas on imaging. Histologically, they are identical to their extracranial counterpart, with sheets and/or nodules of pale histiocytes admixed with a mixed inflammatory infiltrate, variable fibrosis and emperipolesis. The neoplastic histocytes are typically positive for CD68, CD11c and S-100 and negative for CD1a and langerin. This chapter will review the clinical and pathologic features of this rare lymphohistocytic lesion.

Chapter 4 - Angiocentric gliomas are a relatively recently recognized tumor entity, first described by two different groups, Wang and coworkers and Lellouch-Tubiana and colleagues, both in 2005. They are considered low grade tumors (World Health Organization grade I neoplasms) which most commonly arise in pediatric patients in superficial cerebrocortical locations. Most patients present with epilepsy. The tumor is marked by characteristic monomorphic appearing bipolar spindled cells which arrange themselves around cortical blood vessels. The tumor often has an infiltrative margin and evidence of subpial aggregation of cells may be present. Features of high grade tumors, such as prominent mitotic activity, necrosis or vascular proliferation, are usually absent. Similar to other pharmacoresistent epilepsy associated tumors, a subset of these lesions have also been described as having adjacent focal cortical dysplasia. Similar to other gliomas, angiocentric gliomas usually stain with glial markers such as glial fibrillary acidic protein (GFAP) and S-100 protein. Recent work has noted that MYB-QKI fusions are a highly specific and sensitive genetic finding in angiocentric gliomas. The tumor has a generally favorable prognosis and most are cured by surgical resection. This chapter will review the clinical and pathologic features of this relatively rare central nervous system neoplasm.

Chapter 5 - Chordoid gliomas (CG) are rare neoplasms of the central nervous system that arise from the roof or the anterior wall of the third ventricle and are more common in middle-aged females. CG are non-invasive and can be asymptomatic or present with non-specific neurological symptoms that vary depending on size and location of the tumor. On magnetic resonance imaging (MRI), CG appear as a well-circumscribed tumor with a round or an oval shape. Chordoid glioma was first described in 1995 and was later classified as a grade II neoplasm by the World Health Organization (WHO). Morphologically, the tumor is marked by a proliferation of cohesive clusters of epithelioid cells with prominent eosinophilic cytoplasm and a vacuolated appearing, mucin-rich stroma. The tumor is typically accompanied by a lymphoplasmacytic infiltrate with Russell bodies. CG stain with antibodies to glial fibrillary acidic protein (GFAP), CD34, and thyroid transcription factor 1 (TTF-1). It has been variously hypothesized that CG originate from glial ependymal cells or from the organum vasculosum. Tumor-directed surgery is the mainstay of treatment of GC. Most tumors do well clinically upon gross total resection; however, cases will recur if not completely resected and can cause complications and death related to tumor location. In this chapter, the authors will review the histological and clinical features of chordoid gliomas.

Chapter 6 - Dysplastic cerebellar gangliocytomas, also referred to as Lhermitte-Duclos disease, are rare low grade tumors of the cerebellar hemisphere that were first described in 1920. Most cases present in adulthood and the lesion is associated with PTEN mutations and Cowden syndrome. They typically present with signs and symptoms of mass effect, obstructive hydrocephalus and increased intracranial pressure. On imaging studies, they appear as distortions of the cerebellar hemispheric architecture with enlarged cerebellar folia and sometimes cystic changes. Histologically, they are marked by an abnormal collection of large ganglionic cells. There is no evidence of a glioma component in these lesions, such as one might see in a ganglioglioma. Mitotic activity, necrosis or vascular proliferative changes are not typically seen. The ganglion cells stain with immunomarkers typically used to highlight neuronal cells, such as synaptophysin. Surgical resection is curative in the majority of cases, but local recurrence may be encountered in a subset of cases. Patients should be followed for other manifestations of Cowden syndrome.

Chapter 7 - Cerebellar liponeurocytoma is a rare cerebellar tumor which is marked by admixed neurocytic and lipoma-like components. The lesion is thought to arise from cerebellar progenitor cells. Most patients are adults and the tumor shows no gender predilection. Patients typically present with symptoms of headaches, ataxia, gait disturbances, and signs related to increased intracranial pressure. Histologically, the tumor is marked by sheets of uniformly appearing, rounded cells with intermixed lipid-rich cells. Features typically associated with high grade tumors, such as prominent mitotic activity, necrosis and vascular proliferation, are usually absent. The neurocytic cells typically stain with markers of neuronal differentiation including neuron specific enolase, synaptophysin and MAP-2. Ki-67 cell proliferation indices are typically low, generally in the range of 1-3%. TP53 missense mutations have been noted in about 20% of tumors. Cerebellar liponeurocytomas are considered World Health Organization (WHO) grade II neoplasms. Most patients have a favorable prognosis, with survival in excess of 5 years. A subset of tumors do recur and recurrent tumors may show evidence of increased mitotic figures, necrosis or vascular proliferation. This chapter will review the clinicopathologic features of these neoplasms.

In: Tumors of the Central Nervous System ISBN: 978-1-53619-628-3
Editor: James A. Reed © 2021 Nova Science Publishers, Inc.

Chapter 1

EMBRYONAL TUMOR WITH MULTILAYERED ROSETTES, C19MC-ALTERED

Emad Ababneh, MD and Richard Prayson[*], *MD, MEd*

Department of Anatomic Pathology, Cleveland Clinic,
Cleveland, OH, US

ABSTRACT

Embryonal Tumor with Multilayered Rosettes (EMTR) is an aggressive, WHO grade IV tumor. It was defined as a distinct entity in the most recent WHO classification of tumors of the brain and spinal cord in 2016. Previously, it was diagnosed under the umbrella of the primitive neuroectodermal tumors (PNET) family with heterogeneous morphological patterns of medulloepithelioma, ependymoblastoma, and embryonal tumor with abundant neuropil and true rosettes. The growing evidence that this group of tumors shares the characteristic chromosome 19 miRNA cluster (*C19MC*) amplification as well as their distinct clinical behavior made the creation of this entity possible. The diagnosis of this entity is still challenging to make, whether for its rarity or the overlapping histology and clinical features with other embryonal tumors. Furthermore, the ongoing discovery of further genetic driving events, for instance,

---

[*] Corresponding Author's E-mail: praysor@ccf.org.

DICER1 mutations, may lead to refinements in the prognosis and potential therapy. In this chapter, we are going to discuss this entity in detail, reviewing the clinical, pathological, molecular and prognostic features of this rare entity.

INTRODUCTION

Embryonal tumors of the central nervous system are rare aggressive neoplasms. They are mainly pediatric neoplasms, representing 10-15% of primary pediatric brain tumors while only representing <1% of primary brain tumors in adults. Medulloblastoma is by far the predominant tumor type in this group with all non-medulloblastoma embryonal tumors representing up to 2% or less of all childhood brain tumors [1].

The 2016 World Health Organization (WHO) classification of central nervous tumors (CNS) refined the entities within the embryonal tumor category with more emphasis on molecular subtyping [2]. Entities such as ependymoblastoma and embryonal tumor with abundant neuropil and true rosettes (ETANTR), as well as a subset of medulloepitheliomas were grouped together after the discovery of a shared chromosome 19 miRNA cluster (*C19MC*) amplification and similar clinical behavior [2-4]. A new entity termed embryonal tumor with multilayered rosettes (EMTR), *C19MC*-altered (EMTR-C19MC altered) was created [2]. This change also accompanied the disappearance of the umbrella term of primitive neuroectodermal tumors (PNETs) that used to include these various tumor subtypes [2, 5].

ERANTR was first formally described by Eberhart et al. in 2000 as a tumor with distinctive histological features within the PNET family [6]. It was histologically distinguished from other PNETs by virtue of its rich paucicellular fibrillar neuropil matrix and the presence of true rosettes with well-formed lumens [6]. Case reports describing this entity started to appear in the literature, yet the 2007 WHO classification of CNS tumors did not recognize it as a distinct entity [5].

Ependymoblastoma, on the other hand, has a more convoluted history as a diagnostic entity. Baily and Cushing, in their 1926 classification of tumors of the glioma group, described two types of ependymal tumors, ependymomas and ependymoblastomas; yet, the non-reproducible feature of "ependymal spongioblasts" in the latter entity, cells with cytoplasmic processes extending toward vessels, failed to have significant correlation with biological behavior. The ependymoblastoma designation was abandoned in favor of the preferred designation as ependymoma [7]. Kernohan et al. in 1938 reintroduced the term after noticing that some ependymomas show more primitive features and suggested they must be arising from ependymoblasts [7]. This distinction also implied that ependymoblastoma designated a more malignant tumor as compared to ependymoma. Rubinstein et al., redefined ependymoblastomas as tumors with predominantly primitive elements, which show focal ependymal differentiation, through the demonstration of ependymoblastic rosettes [8]. When the category of PNET was introduced, proposals were introduced to include ependymoblastoma as type of PNET [9]. This proposal was adopted by the 2000 and 2007 WHO classification schema [5]. The introduction of ERANTR in various reports further complicated the diagnosis of ependymoblastoma, as both entities show primitive cells with "ependymoblastic rosettes" as well as multilayered rosettes, with ERANTRs showing evidence of neuronal differentiation in the form of abundant neuropil.

Medulloepithelioma was described initially by Baily and Cushing in 1926. It is described as the most primitive CNS tumor [10]. A subset of medulloepitheliomas harbor an alteration in *C19MC* microRNA cluster, but a significant proportion of them do not carry this abnormality [11-12]. So, in the 2016 WHO classification of CNS tumors, medulloepitheliomas are still grouped as a distinct entity from EMTR [2]. The current definition of medulloepitheliomas is CNS embryonal tumors with a prominent neuroepithelium that resembles embryonic neural tube in addition to poorly differentiated neuroepithelial cells [2, 10].

In their seminal paper, Korshunov et al. showed that fluorescent in situ hybridization (FISH) analysis disclosed amplification of 19q13.42 locus (covering the *C19MC* genomic locus) in majority of embryonal tumors showing ependymoblastic rosettes with an even distribution between

ETANRs and ependymoblastomas [4]. In a subsequent study, they also demonstrated this abnormality in a cohort of cases including medulloepitheliomas [11]. They also showed similar clinical parameters between the different histological variants, further advocating for their proposed single entity of EMTR, *C19MC*-altered [11], a designation subsequently adopted by the 2016 WHO classification of tumors of the CNS [2].

CLINICAL PRESENTATION

As discussed earlier, EMTR is primarily a tumor of childhood, with most tumors arising in patients less than 4 years of age [11, 13]. Despite that, it remains one of the rarest primary brain tumors to occur, representing less than 1% of primary tumors of the CNS even in this age group. They show a similar distribution among males and females, with slight female predominance reported in some series [14]. EMTRs most commonly arise in the cerebral hemispheres; nevertheless, they have been reported in various locations both in the supra- and infratentorial compartments, with rare cases reported in the spinal cord [12].

Similar to other brain tumors, the initial presentation is heterogenous and depends on tumor location [12, 15]. Signs and symptoms of increased intracranial pressure, such as headache, nausea, vomiting and visual disturbances are among the common presenting symptoms [13, 16]. Confusion, seizures and other motor impairment, such as torticollis, have also been reported [16].

Magnetic resonance imaging (MRI) findings are similar to those of other embryonal tumors with an overall larger size (in some reports up to 8 cm) [13, 17]. They show variable (heterogenous) signal patterns and frequently show diffusion restriction [13, 17-18]. Overall, they appear well-demarcated, exhibit mass effect without edema, and demonstrate heterogeneous contrast enhancement [18]. A cystic component and intramural hemorrhage have been reported as well [19].

A subset of EMTR show a *DICER1* mutation, which can be associated with *DICER1* predisposition syndrome [12]. This rare association and syndrome can predispose patients to a variety of benign and malignant tumors in different organs including lungs, thyroid, ovary as well as the CNS. In an overlapping age group with EMTR, pleuropulmonary blastoma, cystic nephroma and pineoblastoma are examples of *DICER1* predisposition syndrome associated tumors [20].

PATHOLOGIC FEATURES

EMTRs show histopathology features shared across embryonal tumors of the CNS including hypercellularity with round to oval crowded nuclei with generally stippled chromatin. These tumors tend to show brisk mitotic activity, frequent apoptotic bodies, and variable degree of pleomorphism [21-22].

EMTRs classically have a biphasic appearance of cellular unstructured primitive areas (Figure 1) and paucicellular fibrillary neuropil rich areas (Figure 2) [11-13, 21]. Multilayered rosettes with true lumens are found in most cases but can be focal and inconspicuous (Figure 3). The true lumen of the rosette can be small and round or large and slit like with occasional intraluminal debris (Figure 4). The rosettes can arise abruptly in the hypocellular neuropil rich areas. Ganglion cells may be present in neuropil rich areas.

EMTRs have heterogeneous morphologies, as they currently encompass tumors formerly classified as ependymoblastomas and medulloepithelioma [12, 22]. So, a subset of cases lacks the neuropil areas and are mostly composed of primitive cells with multilayered rosettes (formerly classified as ependymoblastoma). Yet another histologic variation is that of medulloepithelioma, which a minor subset of it falls under ETMR, and they show primitive neural tube-like morphology with tubular, trabecular and papillary patterns and lack the true rosettes and neurocytic and gangliocytic differentiation of fibrillary neuropil areas and ganglion cells.

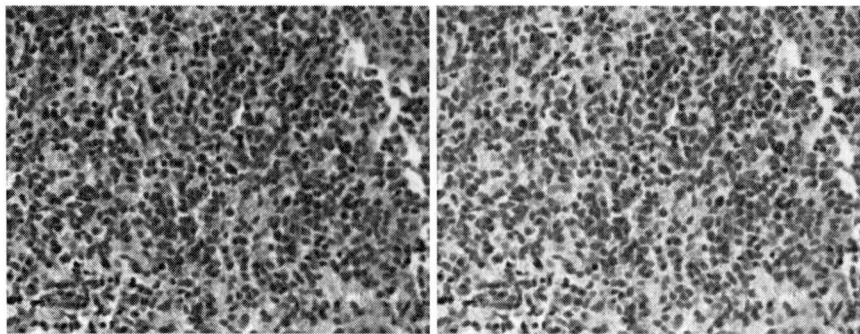

Figure 1. This case of EMTR shows hypercellular areas of primitive looking cells with high nuclear: cytoplasmic ratio, a finding common to most embryonal tumors (hematoxylin and eosin, original magnification 200X).

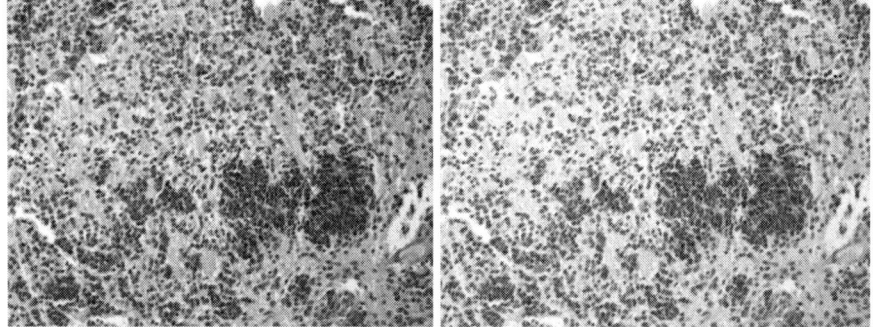

Figure 2. EMTRs show biphasic morphology of hypercellular immature cells with areas of paucicellular neuropil rich morphology. Few multilayered rosettes can be seen in the lower left corner (hematoxylin and eosin, original magnification 200X).

ANCILLARY STUDIES

EMTRs show a variable pattern of reactivity to a number of antibodies, depending on different morphologic elements. The neuropil rich areas show diffuse positivity for neural markers like synaptophysin (Figure 5), NeuN and neurofilament proteins [12-13, 21-22]. Focal to patchy staining for glial fibrillary acidic protein (GFAP) can be found in some cases [13]. The more immature or rosette areas show variable expression of epithelial membrane antigen (EMA), cytokeratin and CD99. In contrast to some other embryonal tumors, INI-1 is retained and diffusely positive. In the study by Korshunov et al., gene expression profile identified LIN28A as a specific marker for ETMR; they showed that LIN28A specific antibodies are reactive in all cases of ETMR, with only rare focal staining noted in other tumors [23]. This makes LIN28A a highly sensitive and specific immunohistochemical stain in the diagnosis of ETMRs. Although it has limited diagnostic utility, the apical regions of the tumor cells in the rosettes' lumen can contain CD99 or D2-40 positive basal bodies of cilia.

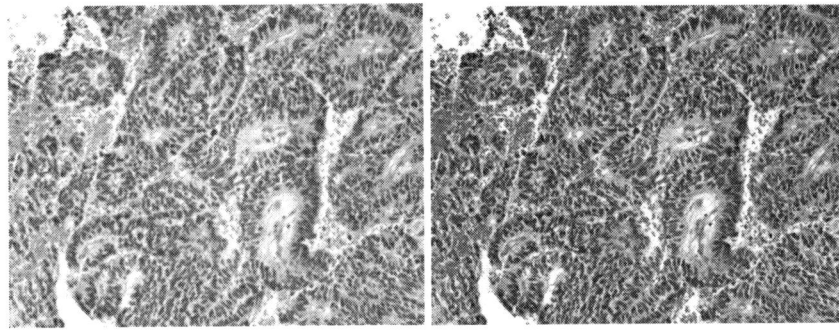

Figure 3. The characteristic "ependymoblastic" rosettes with multilayered growth of primitive looking cells and true lumen. Sometimes the rosettes are only focally present (hematoxylin and eosin, original magnification 200X).

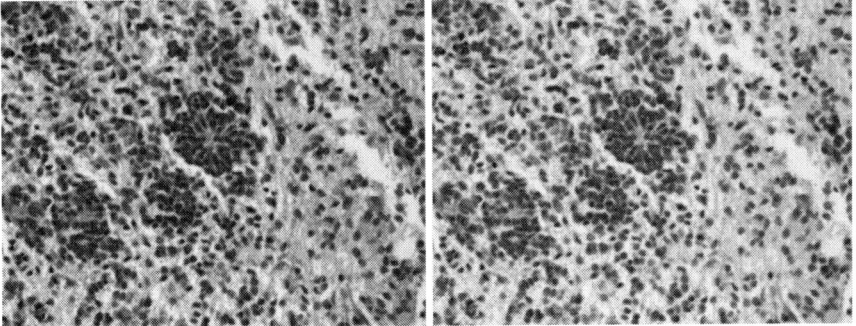

Figure 4. Occasionally the lumen of the rosettes show intraluminal debris (hematoxylin and eosin, original magnification 400X).

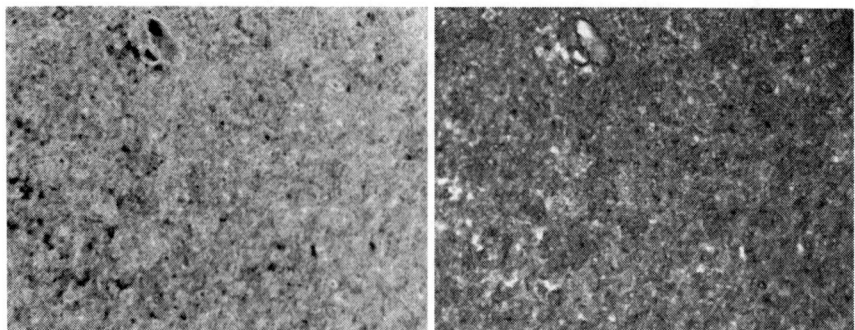

Figure 5. Synaptophysin is diffusely positive, especially in neuropil rich cases (original magnification 200X).

MOLECULAR FINDINGS

The main molecular finding of EMTR is amplification of 19q13.42 locus (*C19MC* genomic locus). This genomic alteration was first noted into as a novel finding in one case of a tumor under the prior name of embryonal tumor with abundant neuropil and true rosettes (ETANTR) by Pfister et al. [3]. Subsequently, in a study by Li et al., this alteration was described in subset of aggressive PNETs of the CNS [24]. The 19q13.42 locus harbors a large cluster of miRNAs; their function is yet to be fully understood but under normal condition, they show restricted expression in undifferentiated and germinal tissues such as placenta and testes [24]. Reports have indicated a role in cellular differentiation and they appear to be regulated by other transcriptional regulators of embryonic stem cells multilineage differentiation potency. This potentially suggests a possible role in altering the response of the neural tissue precursor response to differentiation and survival signals [24].

In their seminal paper, Korshunov et al. showed that virtually all of the ETANTRs and ependymoblastomas in their study consistently demonstrated evidence of a *C19MC* amplification [4]. They confirmed this finding in another subsequent paper which also showed this distinctive alteration in embryonal tumors with medulloepithelioma histologic features [11].

Two points are worth noting here. First, only a subset of medulloepitheliomas show alteration in C19MC, which explains why the 2016 WHO classification of CNS tumors still has a distinct category for medulloepitheliomas, reserved for cases without the C19MC alteration [22]. The other point is that although *C19MC* amplification is the hallmark of ETMR, it is only present in 90% of the cases. The remaining 10% of cases have amplification of another miRNA cluster on chromosome 13 (*MIR17HG*), which is also reported concurrent with C19MC [12, 25]. More common than *MIR17HG* amplification is biallelic mutations of *DICER1*, which is mutually exclusive from *C19MC* and *MIR17HG* amplifications [12, 25]. *DICER1* mutational patterns in these cases are similar to what is seen in other *DICER1* predisposition syndrome related tumors. The available literature suggests that EMTRs with these different driver mutations show a similar downstream molecular profile and are biologically related [25]. This is in contrast to *C19MC* negative medulloepitheliomas, which seem to be molecularly distinct from EMTRs [12].

DIFFERENTIAL DIAGNOSIS

The main differential diagnoses of EMTR are the other embryonal tumors of the CNS, as they show similar age distribution and mostly show atypical primitive cells with brisk mitotic activity and tumor cells with a high nuclear/cytoplasmic ratio. Embryonal tumors with histologic features of medulloepithelioma but lack the *C19MC* alteration should be diagnosed as medulloepithelioma per the WHO.

Medulloblastoma is the most common among the embryonal tumors. Similar to EMTR, it occurs predominantly in the pediatric population [1]. Medulloblastomas most commonly arise in the cerebellum in contrast to the predominantly cerebral location of EMTRs. They have little, if any, neuropil, except in the nodular type. The hallmark rosettes found in medulloblastoma are neuroblastic (Homer-Wright) pseudorosettes which lack true lumens and perivascular pseudorosettes, unlike EMTRs which show multilayered rosettes with true lumens and rarely show a perivascular growth pattern. Medulloblastomas are negative for LIN28A which is highly specific for EMTR and they do not show the characteristic *C19MC* amplification [23].

Atypical teratoid/rhabdoid tumor (AT/RT) is an embryonal tumor that needs to be excluded when encountering a case of EMTR, as it can rarely have ependymoblastic rosettes. It mainly affects patients below 2 years of age and is evenly distributed between infratentorial and supratentorial locations. AT/RTs invariably show rhabdoid cells at least focally. Rhabdoid cells have round eccentric nuclei with open chromatin, prominent nucleoli and sometimes show eosinophilic cytoplasmic inclusions. The most important ancillary study for the diagnosis of AT/RTs is the loss of INI-1 expression, which is retained in virtually all EMTRs [26]. The use of LIN28A in this differential diagnosis should be evaluated with caution, as up to 20% of AT/RTs, according to some reports, can show focal reactivity [27]. *C19MC* amplification is absent in AT/RTs.

Lastly, as EMTRs show well-formed true rosettes, they should not be confused with ependymoma, especially anaplastic ependymomas. Ependymomas have a different biology, behavior and outcome. True, well-formed rosettes are typical of low grade well-differentiated ependymoma and occur in much lower frequency in anaplastic ependymomas. The rosettes in ependymomas show a single layer of mitotically inactive cells lining the lumen, in contrast to the multilayered, primitive looking, briskly mitotic cells lining the lumens in the rosettes of EMTRs. Despite the prior terminology for some of EMTR cases as ependymoblastoma, these tumors are not "primitive ependymomas" but rather are embryonal tumors that characterized by rosettes with some "ependymal" differentiation. Ependymomas are diffusely positive for GFAP, focally positive for synaptophysin and other neural markers, negative for LIN28A, and do not show amplification of C19MC [23, 27]; a profile that is quite different from EMTRs.

PROGNOSIS AND TREATMENT

The prognosis of EMTRs remains dismal with a 5-year survival rates below 30%. Reports of long-term survivors exist, yet this is the exception rather than the rule [12-14]. Due to the rarity of the tumor, enough data to help build a standardized treatment plans is lacking. Surgical resection might be an option, especially with a localized disease. The acute presentation of large tumor size, as well as the fact that most patients are below 2 years old, make resection challenging with a risk for high-risk of perioperative complications [14]. No specific chemotherapeutic regimens have been studied for EMTRs in particular and current data are driven by clinical trials for CNS "PNETs" and other high risk embryonal tumors [12]. Few reports showed survival benefits with the addition of radiotherapy to treatment regimens, yet it is not commonly attempted [14]. This is due to the lack of standard protocols and the risk for high radiation toxicity and side effects especially to the vulnerable age group EMTRs patients. The discovery of a link between *C19MC* amplification, overexpression of LIN28 and the activation of the mammalian target of rapamycin (*mTOR*) pathway is paving the way for agents such as decitabine and actinomycin D, as well as targeted mTOR pathway inhibitors, like rapamycin [12, 28-29]. Although it is challenging for an individual trial to have sufficient numbers of EMTR cases, the current of presence multiple clinical trials investigating a number of these new drugs in pediatric brain tumors (e.g., ClinicalTrials.gov Identifiers NCT01294670, NCT00867178, NCT01076530, NCT00994500) provides hope for more understanding and data to help patients with EMTR.

REFERENCES

[1]   Ostrom QT, Gittleman H, Truitt G, et al. CBTRUS statistical report: Primary brain and other central nervous system tumors diagnosed in

the United States in 2011-2015. *Neuro-Oncol.* 2018;20(S4): 1-86 iv1-iv86. doi:10.1093/neuonc/noy131.

[2] Louis DN, Perry A, Reifenberger G, et al. The 2016 World Health Organization classification of tumors of the central nervous system: a summary. *Acta Neuropathol.* 2016;131(6):803-820. doi:10.1007/s00401-016-1545-1.

[3] Pfister S, Remke M, Castoldi M, et al. Novel genomic amplification targeting the microRNA cluster at 19q13.42 in a pediatric embryonal tumor with abundant neuropil and true rosettes. *Acta Neuropathol.* 2009;117(4):457-464. doi:10.1007/s00401-008-0467-y.

[4] Korshunov A, Remke M, Gessi M, et al. Focal genomic amplification at 19q13.42 comprises a powerful diagnostic marker for embryonal tumors with ependymoblastic rosettes. *Acta Neuropathol.* 2010;120(2):253-260. doi:10.1007/s00401-010-0688-8.

[5] Louis DN, Ohgaki H, Wiestler OD, et al. The 2007 WHO classification of tumours of the central nervous system. *Acta Neuropathol.* 2007;114(2):97-109. doi:10.1007/s00401-007-0243-4.

[6] Eberhart CG, Brat DJ, Cohen KJ, et al. Pediatric neuroblastic brain tumors containing abundant neuropil and true rosettes. *Pediatr. Dev. Pathol.* 2000;3(4): 346-352. doi:10.1007/s100249910049.

[7] Judkins AR, Ellison DW. Ependymoblastoma: dear, damned, distracting diagnosis, farewell! *Brain Pathol.* 2010;20(1):133-139. doi:10.1111/j.1750-3639.2008.00253.x.

[8] Rubinstein LJ. The definition of the ependymoblastoma. *Arch. Pathol.* 1970;90(1): 35-40.

[9] Becker LE, Hinton D. Primitive neuroectodermal tumors of the central nervous system. *Hum. Pathol.* 1983;14(6):538-550. doi:10.1016/ S0046-8177(83)80006-9.

[10] Molloy PT, Yachnis AT, Rorke LB, et al. Central nervous system medulloepithelioma: a series of eight cases including two arising in the pons. *J. Neurosurg.* 1996;84(3):430-436. doi:10.3171/jns.1996.84.3.0430.

[11] Korshunov A, Sturm D, Ryzhova M, et al. Embryonal tumor with abundant neuropil and true rosettes (ETANTR), ependymoblastoma,

and medulloepithelioma share molecular similarity and comprise a single clinicopathological entity. *Acta Neuropathol.* 2014; 128(2):279-289. doi:10.1007/s00401-013-1228-0.

[12] Lambo S, von Hoff K, Korshunov A, Pfister SM, Kool M. ETMR: a tumor entity in its infancy. *Acta Neuropathol.* 2020;140(3):249-266. doi:10.1007/s00401-020-02182-2.

[13] Gessi M, Giangaspero F, Lauriola L, et al. Embryonal tumors with abundant neuropil and true Rosettes: A distinctive CNS primitive neuroectodermal tumor. *Am. J. Surg. Pathol.* 2009;33(2):211-217. doi:10.1097/PAS.0b013e318186235b.

[14] Jaramillo S, Grosshans DR, Philip N, et al. Radiation for ETMR: Literature review and case series of patients treated with proton therapy. *Clin. Transl. Radiat. Oncol.* 2019;15:31-37. doi:10.1016/j.ctro.2018.11.002.

[15] Pagès M, Masliah-Planchon J, Bourdeaut F. Embryonal tumors of the central nervous system. *Curr. Opin. Oncol.* 2020;32(6):623-630. doi:10.1097/CCO.0000000000000686.

[16] Horwitz M, Dufour C, Leblond P, et al. Embryonal tumors with multilayered rosettes in children: the SFCE experience. *Child's Nerv. Syst.* 2016;32(2): 299-305. doi:10.1007/s00381-015-2920-2.

[17] Gogia B, Fuller G, Ketonen L. Embryonal tumor with multilayered rosettes (ETMR): clinical, radiological and pathological summary of 6 cases and review of this recently defined C19MC-altered entity (P3.276). *Neurology.* 2016;86(16 Supplement):P3.276. http://n.neurology.org/content/86/16_Supplement/P3.276.abstract.

[18] Wang B, Gogia B, Fuller GN, et al. Embryonal tumor with multilayered rosettes, C19MC-altered: clinical, pathological, and neuroimaging findings. *J. Neuroimaging.* 2018;28(5): 483-489. doi:10.1111/ jon.12524.

[19] Pei YC, Huang GH, Yao XH, et al. Embryonal tumor with multilayered rosettes, C19MC-altered (ETMR): A newly defined pediatric brain tumor. *Int. J. Clin. Exp. Pathol.* 2019;12(8): 3156-3163. www.ijcep.com/.

[20] Schultz KAP, Rednam SP, Kamihara J, et al. PTEN, DICER1, FH, and their associated tumor susceptibility syndromes: Clinical features, genetics, and surveillance recommendations in childhood. *Clin. Cancer Res.* 2017;23(12): e76-e82. doi:10.1158/1078-0432.CCR-17-0629.

[21] Blessing MM, Alexandrescu S. Embryonal tumors of the central nervous system: An update. *Surg. Pathol. Clin.* 2020;13(2):235-247. doi:10.1016/j.path.2020.01.003.

[22] Louis DN, Perry A, Reifenberger G, et al. The 2016 World Health Organization classification of tumors of the central nervous system: a summary.*Acta Neuropathol.*2016;131(6):803-820. doi:10.1007/s00401-016-1545-1.

[23] Korshunov A, Ryzhova M, Jones DTW, et al. LIN28A immunoreactivity is a potent diagnostic marker of embryonal tumor with multilayered rosettes (ETMR). *Acta Neuropathol.* 2012;124(6):875-881. doi:10.1007/s00401-012-1068-3.

[24] Li M, Lee KF, Lu Y, et al. Frequent amplification of a chr19q13.41 microRNA polycistron in aggressive primitive neuroectodermal brain tumors. *Cancer Cell.* 2009;16(6):533-546. doi:10.1016/j.ccr.2009.10.025.

[25] Lambo S, Gröbner SN, Rausch T, et al. The molecular landscape of ETMR at diagnosis and relapse. *Nature.* 2019;576(7786):274-280. doi:10.1038/s41586-019-1815-x.

[26] Judkins AR, Mauger J, Ht A, et al. Immunohistochemical analysis of hSNF5/INI1 in pediatric CNS neoplasms. *Am. J. Surg. Pathol.* 2004;28(5):644-650.https://journals.lww.com/ajsp/Fulltext/ 2004/05000/Immunohistochemical_Analysis_of_hSNF5_ INI1_in.13.aspx.

[27] Rao S, Rajeswarie RT, Chickabasaviah Yasha T, et al. LIN28A, a sensitive immunohistochemical marker for Embryonal tumor with multilayered rosettes (ETMR), is also positive in a subset of Atypical Teratoid/Rhabdoid Tumor (AT/RT). *Child's Nerv. Syst.* 2017;33 (11):1953-1959. doi:10.1007/s00381-017-3551-6.

[28] Spence T, Perotti C, Sin-Chan P, et al. A novel C19MC amplified cell line links Lin28/let-7 to mTOR signaling in embryonal tumor with multilayered rosettes. *Neuro-Oncol.* 2014;16(1):62-71. doi:10.1093/neuonc/not162.

[29] Schmidt C, Schubert NA, Brabetz S, et al. Preclinical drug screen reveals topotecan, actinomycin D, and volasertib as potential new therapeutic candidates for ETMR brain tumor patients. *Neuro-Oncol.* 2017;19(12):1607-1617. doi:10.1093/neuonc/nox093.

In: Tumors of the Central Nervous System
Editor: James A. Reed
ISBN: 978-1-53619-628-3
© 2021 Nova Science Publishers, Inc.

Chapter 2

DYSEMBRYOPLASTIC NEUROEPITHELIAL TUMOR (DNET): A CLINICOPATHOLOGIC REVIEW

Mrinal M. Sarwate, MD and
Richard A. Prayson*, MD, MEd
Cleveland Clinic Department of Anatomic Pathology,
Cleveland, OH, US

ABSTRACT

Dysembryoplastic neuroepithelial tumor (DNET) is a rare low grade (World Health Organization grade I) glioneuronal neoplasm which mostly affects the temporal lobe. It usually presents in the 2nd or 3rd decades of life and is slightly more common in males. Patients with DNET typically present with focal seizures which may be pharmacoresistent and may warrant surgical excision.

---

* Corresponding Author's E-mail: praysor@ccf.org.

On imaging studies, DNET appears to be confined to the cerebral cortex. There may be thickening of the cortex with well demarcated nodules, some showing internal nodularity with a pseudocystic, bubbly appearance due to the mucoid material. Histopathologically, the tumor is composed of oligodendroglial-like cells, patterned intracortical nodules and "floating neurons" seen in the mucoid material. DNET is subdivided into simple and complex variants. The simple variant is composed of specific glioneuronal element only, while the complex variant has glial nodules in addition to specific glioneuronal elements. Coexistent focal cortical dysplasia is a common finding in the adjacent brain tissue. Differential diagnoses of DNET include oligodendroglioma and ganglioglioma. This chapter will review the clinicopathologic features and differential diagnoses of DNET.

History

Dysembryoplastic neuroepithelial tumor (DNET) was first described by Daumas-Duport et al. in 1988 as a tumor seen in patients with medically refractory partial seizures; the report described 39 cases of this entity with clinicopathologic and radiologic correlation and patient follow-up [1]. The tumor they described was intracortical, multinodular, and composed of oligodendrocytes, astrocytes and neurons. Patients typically presented with early onset partial complex seizures. They noted the presence of focal cortical dysplasia in the surrounding tissue and overlying cranial deformities in a subset of cases, which prompted them to use the term "dysembryoplastic," implying a developmental origin. DNET was formally recognized as a distinct entity in the World Health Organization (WHO) Classification of Central Nervous System tumors in 1993 [2].

Demographics

DNET is a rare, WHO grade I glioneuronal neoplasm. It accounts for 1.2% of all central nervous system tumors in people less than 20 years of age, 0.24% of tumors in those above the age of 20 years, and 0.63% of tumors overall across all ages [3]. It usually presents in the 2nd or 3rd decade of life, and is slightly more common in males.

TUMOR LOCALIZATION

Most DNETs are supratentorial in location with a predilection for the temporal lobe. Less commonly, they may arise in the frontal lobe or in other locations [4]. Rarely, DNETs have been reported to involve parietal lobe, occipital lobe, septum pellucidum, caudate nucleus, thalamus, pons, cerebellum, brainstem, and ventricles [4]. Multifocal tumors [5] and familial occurrence [6] of DNET has also been reported in literature.

DNETs have also been reported to occur in patients with neurofibromatosis type 1 (NF1) [7] and XYY syndrome [8]. The exact origin of DNET, as of now, remains unclear; however, they are speculated to have a dysodontogenic or malformative origin [1].

CLINICAL FEATURES

Among patients who undergo neurosurgery for intractable or pharmacoresistent seizures, 17.8-20% are found to have DNET [4]. It is the second most common primary tumor to arise in this clinical setting, following ganglioglioma. In some cases of simple DNET, partial seizures can become secondarily generalized [4]. Other types of seizures that are less commonly seen include generalized tonic-clonic seizures and simple partial seizures. Other than seizures, headaches has been described as a rare symptom in patients with DNET [1]. Neurologic deficits are not commonly seen in DNET. Surgery often is employed for seizure control after many years of symptoms. A 2011 study of 101 cases of DNET showed the mean age of onset of epilepsy to be 9 years and mean age at surgery to be 31 years [9].

RADIOLOGY

On radiologic imaging, DNETs appear to be generally confined to the cerebral cortex. Computed tomography (CT) imaging may show thickening of the cortex with well demarcated nodules and a pseudocystic, bubbly appearance due to the mucoid and microcystic nature of the tumor. Some cases may have low density appearance with focal contrast enhancement, while others may show calcific hyperdensity [1]. However, no mass effect or perilesional edema is seen, which proves important to differentiate DNET from gliomas radiologically. An overlying cranial deformity may be seen in some cases of DNET located on the convexities due to chronic pressure. Magnetic resonance imaging (MRI) studies typically show a well demarcated lesion with a pseudocystic, bubbly appearance with low signal intensity on T1-weighted images and high signal intensity on T2-weighed images.

HISTOPATHOLOGY

DNET is usually a solitary, fairly well demarcated tumor. It is marked by cystic change, and multinodularity. Rarely, tumors may be focally less well demarcated. The bulk of the DNET is intracortical; however, larger tumors may show extension into subcortical white matter [4].

Histologically, characteristic features of DNET are multinodularity and the presence of specific glioneuronal elements consisting of rounded oligodendroglial-like cells with scant cytoplasm and intermixed benign appearing neuronal cells (Figure 1). Special staining for Alcian blue may be useful to highlight the nodularity in a DNET.

DNET is classified into simple and complex subtypes and a controversial "non-specific" subtype. Simple DNET has a "specific glioneuronal element" only, which is composed of columns of axons surrounded by oligodendroglia-like cells, and floating neurons arranged against a mucinous background. The oligodendroglia-like cells may also be arranged in alveolar, microcystic or compact patterns (Figure 2). The floating neurons do not show nuclear atypia or perineuronal satellitosis, and represent normal cortical neurons that are entrapped in the mucinous matrix [4] (Figures 3 & 4). Dysplastic neurons are not seen in DNET.

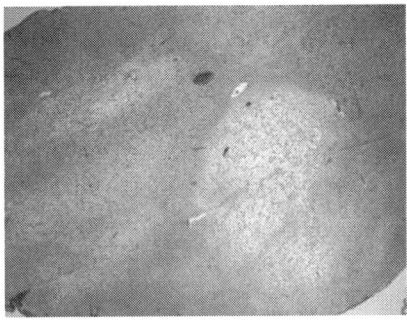

Figure 1. Low magnification appearance of a DNET showing the characteristic multinodular architecture. Most of the nodules are situated primarily in the cortex (hematoxylin and eosin, original magnification 20X).

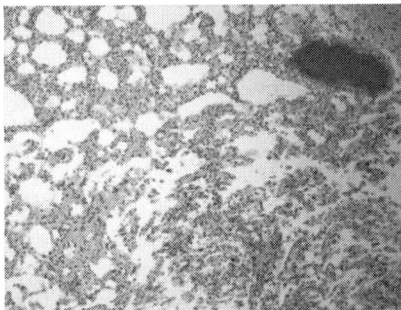

Figure 2. Many of the nodules in a DNET are marked by cells arranged against a microcytic background (hematoxylin and eosin, original magnification 100X).

Complex DNET has glial nodules and perilesional focal cortical dysplasia in addition to specific glioneuronal elements. Glial nodules may morphologically resemble low grade gliomas. Glial nodules may have associated hamartomatous and calcified vasculature. The internodular area may show an abnormal oligodendroglial component [4]. Coexistent focal cortical dysplasia, characterized by architectural disorganization of the adjacent cortex with respect to the neuronal component, is frequently associated with DNET; the focal cortical dysplasia in this setting is classified as Type IIIB in the International League against Epilepsy (ILAE) focal cortical dysplasia classification schema. (Figure 5) Rare complex DNET may show some nuclear atypia, mitosis and microvascular proliferation.

Non-specific DNET is a controversial entity which lacks a specific glioneuronal element, but has glial nodules, and internodular areas similar to complex DNET. Non-specific DNET is diffuse, poorly demarcated, does not have multinodular architecture, and resembles low grade gliomas. Nuclear pleomorphism involving the astrocytic component is not uncommon [4].

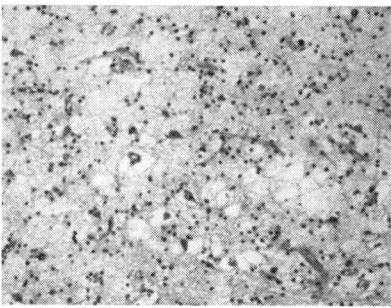

Figure 3. Many of the cells in the nodules have rounded nuclei with scant cytoplasm, resembling oligodendroglial cells. Intermixed are occasional cytologically normal appearing neurons (hematoxylin and eosin, original magnification 200X).

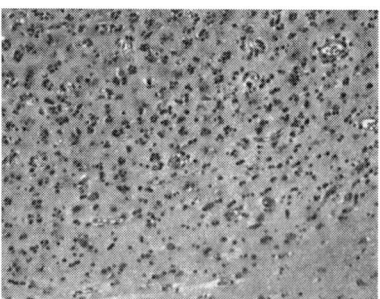

Figure 4. A less microcystic appearing nodule in a DNET (hematoxylin and eosin, original magnification 200X).

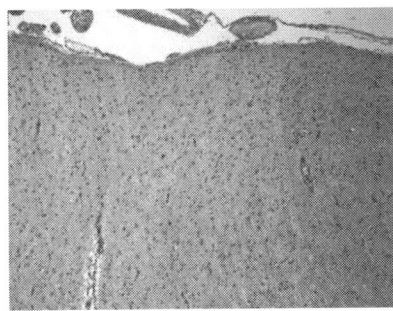

Figure 5. An area of focal cortical dysplasia adjacent to a DNE marked by loss of cortical layer two, a malpositioning of larger 3 neurons where layer 2 normally resides, and molecular layer gliosis (hematoxylin and eosin, original magnification 100X).

Immunohistochemical staining of DNET shows the floating neurons to stain positively for synaptophysin, NeuN, neuron specific enolase, microtubule associated protein 2 (MAP2), and class-III beta-tubulin. Oligodendroglial-like cells are positive for S-100, transcription factor Olig2, myelin-oligodendrocyte glycoprotein and Nogo-A; however, they are negative for glial fibrillary acidic protein (GFAP). Glial nodules may show GFAP positive astrocytes [4]. Nonspecific DNET shows slightly decreased synaptophysin staining with negative staining for all neuronal markers, except MAP2.

A 2011 study of 101 cases of all types of DNET showed CD34 positivity in 61% cases, calbindin positivity in 57%, while nestin positivity was seen in 86% of cases [9]. CD34 positivity is seen in generally peritumoral areas and more commonly in the nonspecific type of DNET. In one study, a BRAF V600E mutation was noted by immunostaining in 30% cases of DNET [10]. BRAF staining, when observed, can be seen in the glial nodules and dysplastic neurons of surrounding focal cortical dysplasia but is absent in the floating neurons. Cell proliferation markers, like Ki-67 or MIB-1, show typically low labelling indices, often less than 3%.

Isocitrate dehydrogenase (IDH)- 1 and -2 mutations and chromosome 1p/19q co-deletion are generally not seen in DNET. These are characteristic findings in oligodendrogliomas, which can look very similar to DNET. However, in a 2011 study of 101 DNETs by Thom et al. an

IDH-1 mutation was noted in 3 cases and 1p/19q co-deletion in another 10 cases (none of which also had an IDH-1 mutation) [9].

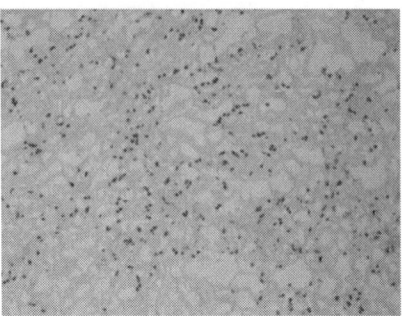

Figure 6. DNET at frozen section. It is usually difficult at the time of frozen section to distinguish a DNET from a microcystic low grade glioma, especially if only a small amount of the tumor is samples (hematoxylin and eosin, original magnification 200X).

On a cytologic squash preparation, DNET shows floating neurons with extracellular mucin and oligodendroglial-like cells. Oligodendroglia-like cells of DNET have larger nuclei as compared to oligodendroglioma cells. They also are marked by nuclear indentation and prominent nucleoli. Oligodendroglioma cells have smooth nuclear contours with rare prominent nucleoli. The background of DNET may show eosinophilic granular bodies [11]. Making a definitive diagnosis at the time of intraoperative consultation may be difficult, unless one can appreciate a multinodular architecture (Figure 6).

DIFFERENTIAL DIAGNOSIS

When formulating a diagnosis of DNET and differentiating it from the common epileptogenic tumors, several things need to be considered. A clinical picture with a history of focal seizures starting early in life and with no progressive neurologic disease should conjure up DNET as a diagnostic possibility. Also, the presence of a temporal lobe, intracortical lesion with no mass effect or peritumoral edema on imaging studies should elicit consideration of DNET.

Simple and complex DNET can be distinguished from ganglioglioma by the absence of perivascular lymphocytic infiltration, absence of prominent neuronal atypia and an absence of a reticulin network within the tumor. DNETs do not contain atypical ganglionic or neuronal cells which are abnormally distributed or clustered, a salient feature of gangliogliomas. Both, nonspecific DNET and ganglioglioma can show CD34 positivity; however, MAP2 positivity is seen only in nonspecific DNET, and not in ganglioglioma. The "glioma" component of the ganglioglioma more commonly resembles an astrocytoma but some gangliogliomas may contain areas that resemble an oligodendroglioma, much like the DNET. A subset of gangliogliomas (anaplastic ganglioglioma) demonstrate features of a higher grade tumor (necrosis, prominent mitotic activity or vascular proliferation), features not typically encountered in a DNET. Rarely, it may be impossible to distinguish between ganglioglioma and DNET or one encounters a tumor which has areas resembling each tumor. These cases can be considered as composite/mixed ganglioglioma and DNET and have been given the name of "composite neuroepithelial tumors" [12] (Figure 7).

Oligodendrogliomas generally are not well demarcated tumors; they typically arise in the white matter and infiltrate to involve the overlying cortex in an expansile fashion. *Perineuronal satellitosis* is noted in oligodendrogliomas and is an infrequent finding in DNETs. MAP 2 expression is useful to differentiate DNET from oligodendroglioma. DNET stains variably and faintly for MAP2, while diffuse oligodendrogliomas show strong perinuclear positivity for MAP2. DNETs do not show concomitant IDH mutations and 1p/19q co-deletions, which is a diagnostic criterion for oligodendroglioma [13]. Some studies have demonstrated utility of BRAF V600E staining in differentiating DNET from oligodendrogliomas [4]. BRAF mutations are more common in DNET than oligodendrogliomas.

Recently, FGFR1 mutations have been found to be positive in a subset of DNETs. A study by Qaddoumi et al. [14] showed FGFR1 mutation in 82% cases of DNET. However, this finding has also been described in a subset of oligodendrogliomas.

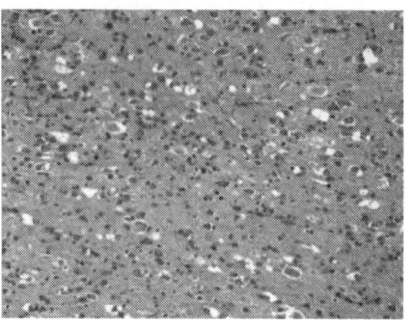

Figure 7. A focal area of a DNET resembling a ganglioglioma, with atypical neuronal cells intermixed with an atypical gliomatous component. Rare cases of so-called composite tumors (ganglioglioma-DNET) have been described (hematoxylin and eosin, original magnification 200X).

TREATMENT AND PROGNOSIS

DNET is a low grade (WHO grade I) glioneuronal tumor with good prognosis following surgical resection. Its circumscription makes it generally amenable to surgical resection. A 2011 study of 101 DNET cases showed that 84% of patients with nonspecific DNET were free of seizures following surgery; 62.5% patients of simple DNET and 53.6% patients with complex DNET were also seizure free [9]. CD34 positive tumors showed better outcome in this study and only one case reportedly showed high grade transformation [9].

Seizure recurrence is usually associated with residual DNET and adjacent focal cortical dysplasia. A study by Chassoux et al. showed complete tumor removal to be the most important factor for obtaining seizure free survival, followed by short epilepsy duration and absence of cortical-subcortical damage at the surgical site [15]. Out of over 1000 cases of DNET reported in literature, only 20 have documented histologic recurrence, and only 6 have been shown to undergo malignant transformation [16]. There are rare reports of high grade astrocytoma arising from a DNET [4]. Anaplastic transformation has been reported after radiation or chemotherapy [17].

CONCLUSION

DNETs are rare tumors, usually encountered in younger patients with medically intractable seizures. DNET, being a low grade tumor, needs to be differentiated from other tumors, particularly oligodendrogliomas, which may have a more aggressive clinical course.

REFERENCES

[1] Daumas-Duport C, Scheithauer BW, Chodkiewicz JP, Laws ER Jr, Vedrenne C. Dysembryoplastic neuroepithelial tumor: a surgically curable tumor of young patients with intractable partial seizures. Report of thirty-nine cases. *Neurosurgery.* 1988 Nov;23(5):545-56. doi: 10.1227/00006123-198811000-00002. PMID: 3143922.

[2] Dozza DC, Rodrigues FF, Chimelli L. Dysembryoplastic neuroepithelial tumor originally diagnosed as astrocytoma and oligodendroglioma. *Arq Neuropsiquiatr.* 2012 Sep;70(9):710-4. doi: 10.1590/s0004-282x2012000900012. PMID: 22990729.

[3] Rosemberg S, Vieira GS. Tumor neuroepitelial disembrioplástico. Estudo epidemiológico de uma única instituição [Dysembryoplastic neuroepithelial tumor. An epidemiological study from a single institution]. *Arq Neuropsiquiatr.* 1998 Jun;56(2):232-6. Portuguese. doi: 10.1590/s0004-282x1998000200011. PMID: 9698733.

[4] Suh YL. Dysembryoplastic neuroepithelial tumors. *J Pathol Transl Med.* 2015 Nov;49(6):438-49. doi: 10.4132/jptm.2015.10.05. Epub 2015 Oct 23. PMID: 26493957; PMCID: PMC4696533.

[5] Leung SY, Gwi E, Ng HK, Fung CF, Yam KY. Dysembryoplastic neuroepithelial tumor. A tumor with small neuronal cells resembling oligodendroglioma. *Am J Surg Pathol.* 1994 Jun;18(6):604-14. PMID: 8179075.

[6] Hasselblatt M, Kurlemann G, Rickert CH, Debus OM, Brentrup A, Schachenmayr W, Paulus W. Familial occurrence of

dysembryoplastic neuroepithelial tumor. *Neurology.* 2004 Mar 23;62(6):1020-1. doi: 10.1212/01.wnl.0000115266.16119.3a. PMID: 15037719.

[7]   Lellouch-Tubiana A, Bourgeois M, Vekemans M, Robain O. Dysembryoplastic neuroepithelial tumors in two children with neurofibromatosis type 1. *Acta Neuropathol.* 1995;90(3):319-22. doi: 10.1007/BF00296517. PMID: 8525807.

[8]   Krossnes BK, Wester K, Moen G, Mørk SJ. Multifocal dysembryoplastic neuroepithelial tumour in a male with the XYY syndrome. *Neuropathol Appl Neurobiol.* 2005 Oct;31(5):556-60. doi: 10.1111/j.1365-2990.2005.00680.x. PMID: 16150126.

[9]   Thom M, Toma A, An S, Martinian L, Hadjivassiliou G, Ratilal B, Dean A, McEvoy A, Sisodiya SM, Brandner S. One hundred and one dysembryoplastic neuroepithelial tumors: an adult epilepsy series with immunohistochemical, molecular genetic, and clinical correlations and a review of the literature. *J Neuropathol Exp Neurol.* 2011 Oct;70(10):859-78. doi: 10.1097/NEN.0b013e3182302475. PMID: 21937911.

[10] Chappé C, Padovani L, Scavarda D, Forest F, Nanni-Metellus I, Loundou A, Mercurio S, Fina F, Lena G, Colin C, Figarella-Branger D. Dysembryoplastic neuroepithelial tumors share with pleomorphic xanthoastrocytomas and gangliogliomas BRAF(V600E) mutation and expression. *Brain Pathol.* 2013 Sep;23(5):574-83. doi: 10.1111/bpa.12048. Epub 2013 Mar 20. PMID: 23442159.

[11] Park JY, Suh YL, Han J. Dysembryoplastic neuroepithelial tumor. Features distinguishing it from oligodendroglioma on cytologic squash preparations. *Acta Cytol.* 2003 Jul-Aug;47(4):624-9. doi: 10.1159/000326579. PMID: 12920757.

[12] Blumcke I, Aronica E, Urbach H, Alexopoulos A, Gonzalez-Martinez JA. A neuropathology-based approach to epilepsy surgery in brain tumors and proposal for a new terminology use for long-term epilepsy-associated brain tumors. *Acta Neuropathol.* 2014 Jul;128(1):39-54. doi: 10.1007/s00401-014-1288-9. Epub 2014 May 25. PMID: 24858213; PMCID: PMC4059966.

[13] Yan H, Parsons DW, Jin G, McLendon R, Rasheed BA, Yuan W, Kos I, Batinic-Haberle I, Jones S, Riggins GJ, Friedman H, Friedman A, Reardon D, Herndon J, Kinzler KW, Velculescu VE, Vogelstein B, Bigner DD. IDH1 and IDH2 mutations in gliomas. *N Engl J Med.* 2009 Feb 19;360(8):765-73. doi: 10.1056/NEJMoa0808710. PMID: 19228619; PMCID: PMC2820383.

[14] Qaddoumi I, Orisme W, Wen J, Santiago T, Gupta K, Dalton JD, Tang B, Haupfear K, Punchihewa C, Easton J, Mulder H, Boggs K, Shao Y, Rusch M, Becksfort J, Gupta P, Wang S, Lee RP, Brat D, Peter Collins V, Dahiya S, George D, Konomos W, Kurian KM, McFadden K, Serafini LN, Nickols H, Perry A, Shurtleff S, Gajjar A, Boop FA, Klimo PD Jr, Mardis ER, Wilson RK, Baker SJ, Zhang J, Wu G, Downing JR, Tatevossian RG, Ellison DW. Genetic alterations in uncommon low-grade neuroepithelial tumors: BRAF, FGFR1, and MYB mutations occur at high frequency and align with morphology. *Acta Neuropathol.* 2016 Jun;131(6):833-45. doi: 10.1007/s00401-016-1539-z. Epub 2016 Jan 25. PMID: 26810070; PMCID: PMC4866893.

[15] Chassoux F, Rodrigo S, Mellerio C, Landré E, Miquel C, Turak B, Laschet J, Meder JF, Roux FX, Daumas-Duport C, Devaux B. Dysembryoplastic neuroepithelial tumors: an MRI-based scheme for epilepsy surgery. *Neurology.* 2012 Oct 16;79(16):1699-707. doi: 10.1212/WNL.0b013e31826e9aa9. Epub 2012 Oct 3. PMID: 23035071.

[16] Chao L, Tao XB, Jun YK, Xia HH, Wan WK, Tao QS. Recurrence and histological evolution of dysembryoplastic neuroepithelial tumor: A case report and review of the literature. *Oncol Lett.* 2013 Oct;6(4):907-914. doi: 10.3892/ol.2013.1480. Epub 2013 Jul 22. PMID: 24137435; PMCID: PMC3796405.

[17] Rushing EJ, Thompson LD, Mena H. Malignant transformation of a dysembryoplastic neuroepithelial tumor after radiation and chemotherapy. *Ann Diagn Pathol.* 2003 Aug;7(4):240-4. doi: 10.1016/s1092-9134(03)00070-4. PMID: 12913847.

In: Tumors of the Central Nervous System ISBN: 978-1-53619-628-3
Editor: James A. Reed © 2021 Nova Science Publishers, Inc.

Chapter 3

ROSAI-DORFMAN DISEASE OF THE CENTRAL NERVOUS SYSTEM

Ahmed Bakhshwin, MD and *Richard A. Prayson*[*], *MD, MEd*
Cleveland Clinic, Department of Anatomic Pathology,
Cleveland, OH, US

ABSTRACT

Rosai-Dorfman disease (RDD) is a rare, benign, idiopathic lymphohistiocytic proliferative disease that has been reported to involve virtually all anatomic sites including, although seldomly, the central nervous system. It tends to present as a solitary mass or as multiple dural masses with a predilection for the cerebral convexities, cavernous sinuses, as well as parasagittal, sellar and suprasellar regions. It is therefore very understandable that these lesions are often thought to be meningiomas on imaging.

---

[*] Corresponding Author's E-mail: praysor@ccf.org.

Histologically, they are identical to their extracranial counterpart, with sheets and/or nodules of pale histiocytes admixed with a mixed inflammatory infiltrate, variable fibrosis and emperipolesis. The neoplastic histocytes are typically positive for CD68, CD11c and S-100 and negative for CD1a and langerin. This chapter will review the clinical and pathologic features of this rare lymphohistocytic lesion.

INTRODUCTION

Sinus histiocytosis with massive lymphadenopathy was first described as a distinct entity in 1969 by Juan Rosai and Ronald Dorfman, hence its designation as Rosai-Dorfman disease (RDD) [1]. It represents a benign histiocytic proliferative disease of uncertain pathogenesis. Typically, the disease presents with painless cervical lymphadenopathy that can be associated with systemic manifestations like fever, anemia, neutrophilia and polyclonal gammopathy [2]. Extranodal involvement has been reported to occur in around 40% of cases [3], with central nervous system (CNS) involvement in less than 5% [4, 5]. The clinical course of RDD is usually indolent and lesions not uncommonly undergo spontaneous regression [6]. To date, recurrent genetic alterations have not been consistently identified and clonality studies have demonstrated polyclonality of the disease in two cases [7].

CLINICAL PRESENTATION

RDD can affect patients over a wide range of ages from 1 to 74 years old; however, it is mostly seen in children and young adults with a mean age of presentation of 20.6 years and with a slight male predominance [8]. Patients with isolated RDD of the CNS tend to be older than those with systemic RDD with a mean age of 39.4 years old [9].

About 5% of RDD involves the CNS [4-5]. Of those, 70% are limited to the CNS with no associated lymphadenopathy or systemic manifestations. Approximately, 75% are intracranial, whereas 25% involve the spine primarily [10]. The leptomeninges is by far the most involved location within the CNS with an over 90% involvement rate [11-13]. As such, on imaging, CNS-RDD often resembles meningioma. However, meningiomas often exhibit higher T2-signal, aiding in separating them from RDD [14]. Both solitary and multiple intracranial RDD have been reported. The clinical symptoms are related to their location. Common symptoms of CNS involvement included headache, nausea and vomiting, seizure, weakness and signs of nerve compression [15-16]. Sellar lesions can present with signs of hypopituitarism and diabetes insipidus [17].

PATHOLOGY

The histomorphologic features of RDD are always consistent, regardless of the location it arises in. RDD is typically marked by sheets or nodules of large, pale histocytes intimately admixed with other inflammatory infiltrates including chiefly lymphocytes and plasma cells (Figures 1, 2). A very helpful clue to the diagnosis, although not a required feature, is the presence of intracytoplasmic lymphocytes and plasma cells consistent with emperipolesis (Figure 3). Intralesional small and intermediate-sized vessels will very commonly demonstrate areas of prominent perivascular chronic inflammation with transmural infiltrates of lymphocytes (Figure 4). By immunohistochemistry, the lesional histiocytes are uniformly positive for both S-100 protein and CD68, while negative for CD1a and langerin (Figures 5, 6).

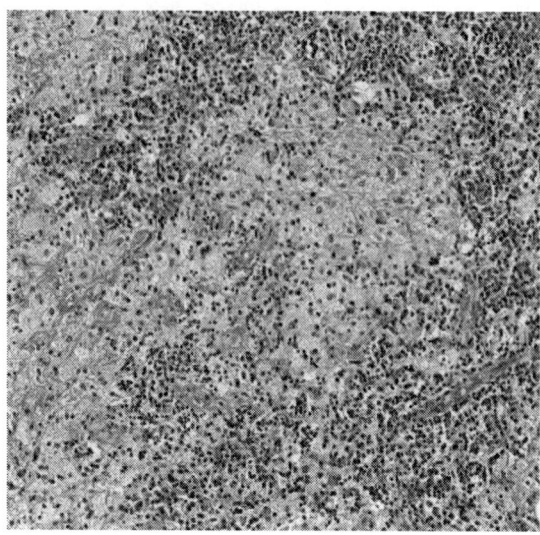

Figure 1. Rosai-Dorfman Disease is marked by sheets of histiocytes with abundant eosinophilic cytoplasm and small, bland nuclei admixed with lymphocytes and plasma cells seen (hematoxylin and eosin, original magnification 100X).

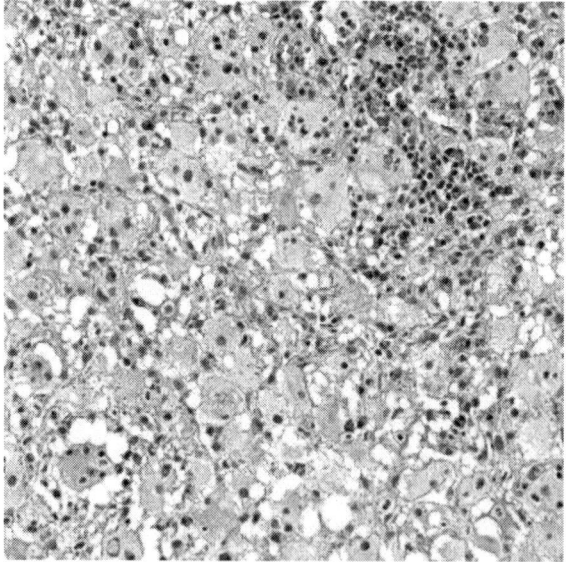

Figure 2. High power view of the lesional histiocytes of Rosai-Dorman Disease (hematoxylin and eosin, original magnification 200X).

Rosai-Dorfman Disease of the Central Nervous System

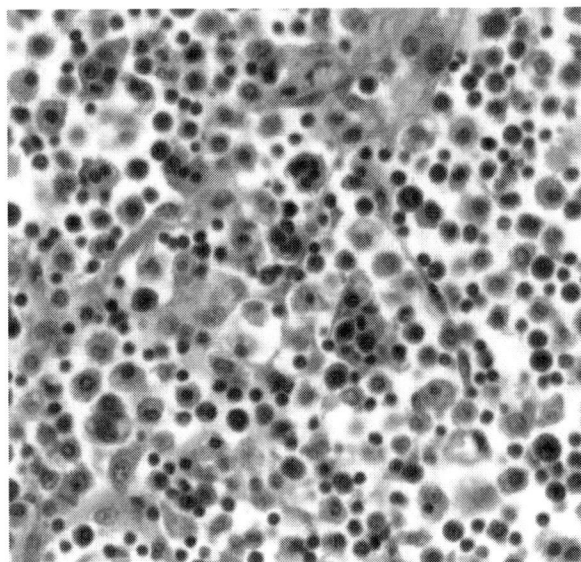

Figure 3. Lymphocytophagocytosis by histiocytes is a common feature of Rosai-Dorfman Disease (hematoxylin and eosin, original magnification 400X).

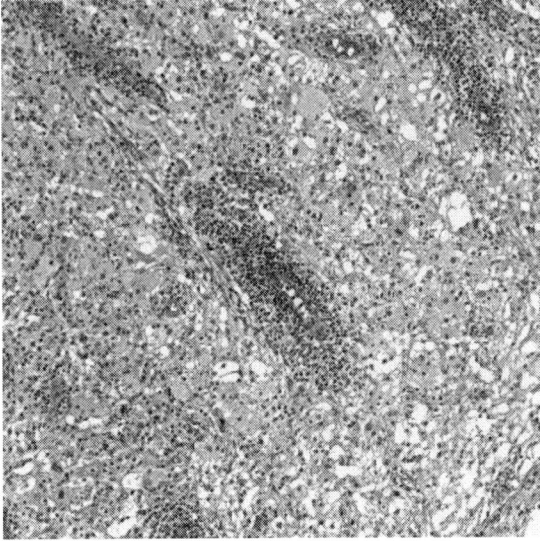

Figure 4. Prominent perivascular condensation of the chronic inflammatory infiltrates is seen (hematoxylin and eosin, original magnification 100X).

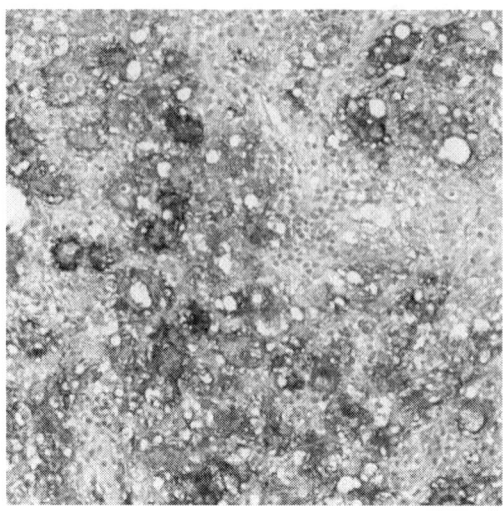

Figure 5. Strong immunoreactivity of the histiocytes in Rosai-Dorfman Disease for S-100 protein (original magnification 200X).

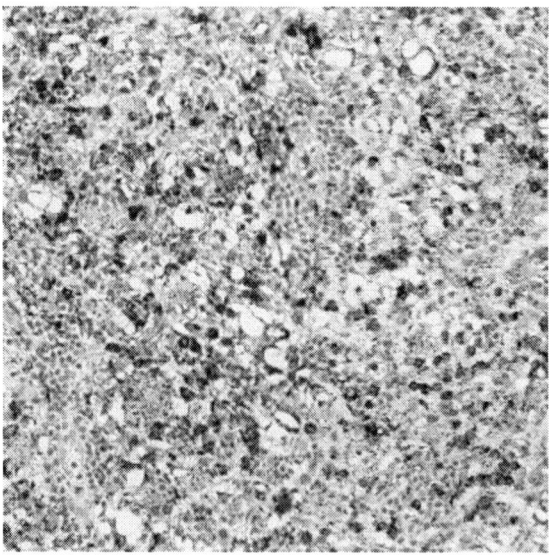

Figure 6. Strong and diffuse positivity of the histocytes for CD68 is noted (original magnification 200X).

DIFFERENTIAL DIAGNOSIS

From an imaging perspective, meningioma is the primary differential diagnostic consideration, given the predilection of RDD to present as a dural-based mass. Most of the histologic variants of meningioma have distinct appearances that are very unlikely to be confused with those of RDD. The only variant that may possess some morphologic overlap is the so-called lymphoplasmacyte-rich meningioma or inflammation-rich meningioma, in which the lesional arachnoid cap cells are obscured by a dense lymphoplasmacytic inflammation. Epithelial membrane antigen (EMA), SSTR2a (somatostatin receptor 2a) and progesterone receptor immunoreactivity can be useful in highlighting tumor cells in meningiomas. This variant has also some unique neuroimaging features. It is frequently associated with peritumoral edema and occasionally involves the meninges in a diffuse "carpet-like" pattern, resembling pachymeningitis [18]. Other tumors that have the propensity to involve the meninges are solitary fibrous tumor and metastasis. These tumors have distinct histomorphologic features that easily separate them apart from RDD.

On the other hand, several histiocytic-rich lesions should be considered, as they share some histologic features with RDD. This includes Langerhans cell histiocytosis (LCH), Erdheim-Chester disease, IgG4-related disease, sarcoidosis and different infectious etiologies. LCH is characterized by sheets of large, oval mononuclear cells with reniform nuclear contours and prominent longitudinal nuclear grooves. It often shows accompanying infiltrates of eosinophils and admixed multinucleated giant cells. The neoplastic cells in LCH are immunoreactive with S-100 protein, CD1a, langerin and BRAF V600E in up to 60% of the cases [19, 20]. The histiocytic cells in RDD are almost invariably negative for CD1a and BRAF V600E.

Like LCH, up to 50% of Erdheim-Chester disease cases harbor a BRAF V600E mutation that can be detected by either immunohistochemistry or other molecular genetic assays like next generation sequencing [21]. The lesional cells of Erdheim-Chester disease are predominantly lipid-laden histocytes with small nuclei and scattered Touton-type multinucleated giant cells. These cells are typically positive for CD68, but negative for CD1a, langerin and S-100 protein.

Demonstration of an increased fraction of IgG4-positive plasma cells in tissue and raised systemic IgG4 levels can help accurately pinpoint IgG4-related disease [22, 23]. While a small number of IgG4-positive plasma cells may be encountered in RDD, numerous IgG4-positive plasma cells (>10/ high power field) favor IgG4-related sclerosing disease. Additional histologic features that are characteristic of IgG-related disease are storiform fibrosis and obliterative phlebitis [24]. The histiocytes of RDD frequently exhibit emperipolesis, a feature that is not typical of IgG4-related disease.

Sarcoidosis is characterized by well-formed non-necrotizing granulomatous inflammation, not typically seen with RDD. Lastly, several infectious etiologies (e.g., mycobacterium and fungal) can be accompanied by a prominent histiocytic inflammatory response that sometimes can be very exuberant and present as inflammatory pseudotumor. Stains for microorganisms (e.g., acid-fast bacteria, Grocott's methenamine silver, and periodic acid-Schiff) can be helpful in identifying the etiology.

TREATMENT

RDD typically pursues a benign clinical course and can spontaneously regress [25]. However, many could persist or even progress. Several treatment modalities have been described including surgery, steroids, and radiation with surgery being the preferred and the most effective among them [26]. That is because surgical resection helps establish the diagnosis and provides rapid improvement of neurologic symptoms. Although not always feasible, complete resection of the mass/masses should be attempted because the extent of the resection is strongly correlated with recurrence rate [27]. In cases with subtotal resection, locations where surgical intervention is challenging, or in relapses, steroid treatment with addition of chemotherapy has resulted in a promising response [28, 29]. Similarly, radiation therapy may be helpful for the same purposes [29, 30].

PATHOGENESIS

Several studies in the literature have attempted to explain the origin of this disease and multiple proposed different theories that could potentially explain the pathogenesis at least to some extent. One group suggested that immune system dysfunction may be the causative factor; they detected human herpesvirus type 6 and Epstein-Barr virus using in situ hybridization in some RDD specimens [31]. Several other groups reported RDD in patients with immunoglobulin G4-related disease, suggesting that the two disorders may have a common pathogenesis [24, 32-34]. Moreover, in patients with familial RDD, SLC29A3 germline mutations have been reported [35-36]. More recently, mutually exclusive KRAS and MAP2K1 mutations have been detected by next-generation sequencing in some patients with RDD [37]. In conclusion, all previously described theories contribute to our understanding of the RDD pathogenesis; nevertheless, the occurrence of RDD cannot be explained by a single theory.

REFERENCES

[1] Rosai J., Dorfman R. F. Sinus histiocytosis with massive lymphadenopathy. A newly recognized benign clinicopathological entity. *Arch. Pathol.* 1969; 87: 63-70.

[2] Vemuganti G. K., Naik M. N., Honavar S. G. Rosai Dorfman disease of the orbit. *J. Hematol. Oncol.* 2008; 1: 7.

[3] Foucar E., Rosai J., Dorfman R., Sinus histiocytosis with massive lymphadenopathy (Rosai-Dorfman disease): review of the entity. *Semin. Diagn. Pathol,* 1990; 7: 19-73.

[4] Andriko J. A., Morrison A., Colegial C. H., Davis B. J., Jones R. V. Rosai-Dorfman disease isolated to the central nervous system: A report of 11 cases. *Mod. Pathol.* 2001; 14: 172-178.

[5] Wu M., Anderson A. E., Kahn L. B. A report of intracranial Rosai-Dorfman disease with literature review. *Ann. Diagn. Pathol.* 2001; 5: 96-102.

[6] Paulli M., Boveri E., Rosso R. Magrini U., Solcia E., Feller A. C., Merz H., Kindl S., Berti E., Facchetti F., Gambini C., Bonetti F., Geerts L., Möller P., Samloff M. Cathepsin D and E co-expression in sinus histiocytosis with massive lymphadenopathy (Rosai-Dorfman disease) and Langerhans' cell histiocytosis: further evidences of a phenotypic overlap between these histiocytic disorders. *Virchows Archiv. A Pathol. Anat.* 1994; 424: 601-606.

[7] Paulli M., Bergamaschi G., Tonon L., Viglio A., Rosso R., Facchetti F., Geerts M. L., Magrini U., Cazzola M. Evidence for a polyclonal nature of the cell infiltrate in sinus histiocytosis with massive lymphadenopathy (Rosai-Dorfman disease). *Br. J. Haematol.* 1995; 91:415-418.

[8] Fukushima T., Yachi K., Ogino A., Ohta T., Watanabe T., Yoshino A., Katayama Y. Isolated intracranial Rosai-Dorfman disease without dural attachment-case report. *Neurol. Med. Chir.* 2011; 51: 136-140.

[9] Kumar R., Singhal U., Kumar Mahapatra A. Intracranial Rosai-Dorfman syndrome: Case Review. *Pan Arab J. Neurosurg.* 2011; 15: 58-63.

[10] Hollowell J. P., Wolfla C. E., Shah N. C., Mark L. P., Whittaker M. H. Rosai-Dorfman disease causing cervical myelopathy. *Spine* (Phila Pa 1976). 2000; 25:1453-1456.

[11] Kattner K. A., Stroink A. R., Roth T. C., Lee J. M. Rosai-Dorfman disease mimicking parasagittal meningioma: case presentation and review of literature. *Surg. Neurol.* 2000; 53: 452-457.

[12] Pauluis W., Perry A., Sahm F. Histiocytic tumors. In: *WHO Classification of Tumours of the Central Nervous System.* (Editors: Louis D. N., Ohgaki H., Wiestler O. D., Cavenee W. K., Ellison D.

W., Figarella-Branger D., Perry A., Reifenberger G., von Deimling A.). IARC. Lyon, FR, 2016. pp. 280-283.

[13] Prayson R. A., Rowe J. J. Dural-based Rosai-Dorfman disease: differential diagnostic considerations. *J. Clin. Neurosci.* 2014; 21: 1872-1873.

[14] Paulli M., Bergamaschi G., Tonon L., Viglio A., Rosso R., Facchetti F., Geerts M. L., Magrini U., Cazzola M. Evidence for a polyclonal nature of the cell infiltrate in sinus histiocytosis with massive lymphadenopathy (Rosai-Dorfman disease). *Br. J. Haematol.* 1995; 91: 415-418.

[15] Tian Y., Wang J., Ge Jz., Ma Z., Ge M. Intracranial Rosai-Dorfman disease mimicking multiple meningiomas in a child: a case report and review of the literature. *Childs Nerv. Syst.* 2015; 31: 317-323.

[16] Mahzoni P., Zavareh M. H., Bagheri M., Hani N., Moqtader B. Intracranial Rosai-Dorfman disease. *J. Res. Med. Sci.* 2012; 17: 304-307.

[17] Jiang Y., Jiang S. Intracranial meningeal Rosai-Dorfman disease mimicking multiple meningiomas: 3 case reports and a literature review. *World Neurosurg.* 2018; 120: 382-390.

[18] Zhu H. D., Xie Q., Gong Y., Mao Y., Zhong P., Hang F. P., Chen H., Zheng M. Z., Tang H. L., Wang D. J., Chen X. C., Zhou L. F. Lymphoplasmacyte-rich meningioma: our experience with 19 cases and a systematic literature review. *Int. J. Clin. Exp. Med.* 2013; 6: 504-515.

[19] Allen C. A., Herad M., McClain L. Langerhans-cell histiocytosis. *N. Engl. J .Med.* 2018; 379: 856-868.

[20] Badalian-Very G, Vergilio JA, Degar BA, MacConaill LE, Brandner B, Calicchio ML, Kuo FC, Ligon AH, Stevenson KE, Kehoe SM, Garraway LA, Hahn WC, Meyerson M, Fleming MD, Rollins BJ. Recurrent BRAF mutations in Langerhans cell histiocytosis. *Blood.* 2010; 116: 1919-1923.

[21] Haroche J., Charlotte F., Arnaud L., von Deimling A., Hélias-Rodzewicz Z., Hervier B., Cohen-Aubart F., Launay D., Lesot A., Mokhtari K., Canioni D., Galmiche L., Rose C., Schmalzing M.,

Croockewit S., Kambouchner M., Copin M. C., Fraitag S., Sahm F., Brousse N., Amoura Z., Donadieu J., Emile J. F. High prevalence of BRAF V600E mutations in Erdheim-Chester disease but not in other non-Langerhans cell histiocytoses. *Blood.* 2012; 120: 2700-2703.

[22] Cheuk W., Chan J. K. IgG4-related sclerosing disease: a critical appraisal of an evolving clinicopathologic entity. *Adv. Anat. Pathol.* 2010; 17: 303-332.

[23] Zhang X., Hyjek E., Vardiman J. A subset of Rosai-Dorfman disease exhibits features of IgG4-related disease. *Am. J. Clin. Pathol.* 2013; 139: 622-632.

[24] Deshpande V., Zen Y., Chan J. K., Yi E. E., Sato Y., Yoshino T., Klöppel G., Heathcote J. G., Khosroshahi A., Ferry J. A., Aalberse R. C., Bloch D. B., Brugge W. R., Bateman A. C., Carruthers M. N., Chari S. T., Cheuk W., Cornell L. D., Fernandez-Del Castillo C., Forcione D. G., Hamilos D. L., Kamisawa T., Kasashima S., Kawa S., Kawano M., Lauwers G. Y., Masaki Y., Nakanuma Y., Notohara K., Okazaki K., Ryu J. K., Saeki T., Sahani D. V., Smyrk T. C., Stone J. R., Takahira M., Webster G. J., Yamamoto M., Zamboni G., Umehara H., Stone J. H. Consensus statement on the pathology of IgG4-related disease. *Mod. Pathol.* 2012; 25: 1181-1192.

[25] Hinduja A., Aguilar L. G., Steineke T., Nochlin D., Landolfi J. C. Rosai-Dorfman disease manifesting as intracranial and intraorbital lesion. *J. Neurooncol.* 2009; 92: 117-20.

[26] Lee-Wing M., Oryschak A., Attariwala G., Ashenhurst M. Rosai-Dorfman disease presenting as bilateral lacrimal gland enlargement. *Am. J. Ophthalmol.* 2001; 131: 677-8.

[27] McPherson C. M., Brown J., Kim A. W., DeMonte F. Regression of intracranial Rosai-Dorfman disease following corticosteroid therapy. Case report *J. Neurosurg.* 2006; 104: 840-844.

[28] Jabali Y., Smrcka V., Pradna J. Rosai-Dorfman disease: successful long-term results by combination chemotherapy with prednisone, 6-mercaptopurine, methotrexate, and vinblastine: a case report. *Int. J. Surg. Pathol.* 2005; 13: 285-289.

[29] McPherson C. M., Brown J., Kim A. W., DeMonte F. Regression of intracranial Rosai-Dorfman disease following corticosteroid therapy. Case report. *J. Neurosurg.* 2006; 104: 840-844.

[30] Kidd D. P., Revesz T., Miller N. R. Rosai-Dorfman disease presenting with widespread intracranial and spinal cord involvement. *Neurology.* 2006; 67:1551-1555.

[31] Levine P. H., Jahan N., Murari P., Manak M., Jaffe E. S. Detection of human herpesvirus 6 in tissues involved by sinus histiocytosis with massive lymphadenopathy (Rosai-Dorfman disease). *J. Infect. Dis.* 1992; 166: 291-295.

[32] Zhang X., Hyjek E., Vardiman J. A subset of Rosai-Dorfman disease exhibits features of IgG4-related disease. *Am. J. Clin. Pathol.* 2013; 139: 622-632.

[33] Kuo T. T., Chen T. C., Lee L. Y., Lu P. H. IgG4-positive plasma cells in cutaneous Rosai-Dorfman disease: an additional immunohistochemical feature and possible relationship to IgG4-related sclerosing disease. *J. Cutan. Pathol.* 2009; 36: 1069-1073.

[34] Chen T. D., Lee L. Y. Rosai-Dorfman disease presenting in the parotid gland with features of IgG4-related sclerosing disease. *Arch Otolaryngol. Head Neck Surg.* 2011; 137: 705-708.

[35] Morgan N. V., Morris M. R., Cangul H., Gleeson D., Straatman-Iwanowska A., Davies N., Keenan S., Pasha S., Rahman F., Gentle D., Vreeswijk M. P., Devilee P., Knowles M. A., Ceylaner S., Trembath R. C., Dalence C., Kismet E., Köseoğlu V., Rossbach H. C., Gissen P., Tannahill D., Maher E. R. Mutations in SLC29A3, encoding an equilibrative nucleoside transporter ENT3, cause a familial histiocytosis syndrome (*Faisalabad histiocytosis*) and familial Rosai-Dorfman disease. *PLoS Genet.* 2010; 6: E1000833.

[36] Melki I., Lambot K., Jonard L., Couloigner V., Quartier P., Neven B., Bader-Meunier B. Mutation in the SLC29A3 gene: a new cause of a monogenic, autoinflammatory condition. *Pediatrics.* 2013; 131: e1308-e1313.

[37] Garces S., Medeiros L. J., Patel K. P., Li S., Pina-Oviedo S., Li J., Garces J. C., Khoury J. D., Yin C. C. Mutually exclusive recurrent KRAS and MAP2K1 mutations in Rosai-Dorfman disease. *Mod. Pathol.* 2017; 30: 1367-1377.

In: Tumors of the Central Nervous System
Editor: James A. Reed

ISBN: 978-1-53619-628-3
© 2021 Nova Science Publishers, Inc.

Chapter 4

THE CLINICAL AND PATHOLOGIC FEATURES OF ANGIOCENTRIC GLIOMA

Richard Prayson[*], *MD, MEd*
Cleveland Clinic Department of Anatomic Pathology,
Cleveland, OH, US

ABSTRACT

Angiocentric gliomas are a relatively recently recognized tumor entity, first described by two different groups, Wang and coworkers and Lellouch-Tubiana and colleagues, both in 2005. They are considered low grade tumors (World Health Organization grade I neoplasms) which most commonly arise in pediatric patients in superficial cerebrocortical locations. Most patients present with epilepsy. The tumor is marked by characteristic monomorphic appearing bipolar spindled cells which arrange themselves around cortical blood vessels. The tumor often has an infiltrative margin and evidence of subpial aggregation of cells may be present. Features of high grade tumors, such as prominent mitotic activity, necrosis or vascular proliferation, are usually absent. Similar to other pharmacoresistent epilepsy associated tumors, a subset of these lesions have also been described as having adjacent focal cortical

---

[*] Corresponding Author's E-mail: praysor@ccf.org.

dysplasia. Similar to other gliomas, angiocentric gliomas usually stain with glial markers such as glial fibrillary acidic protein (GFAP) and S-100 protein. Recent work has noted that MYB-QKI fusions are a highly specific and sensitive genetic finding in angiocentric gliomas. The tumor has a generally favorable prognosis and most are cured by surgical resection. This chapter will review the clinical and pathologic features of this relatively rare central nervous system neoplasm.

INTRODUCTION

The entity of angiocentric glioma was first described in two separate studies that were published in 2005 [1, 2]. Wang and colleagues reported on a series of eight tumors which they termed monomorphous angiocentric glioma [1]. They noted that the tumors had features of both astrocytoma and ependymoma. Five patients were pediatric and all patients presented with epilepsy. They described the tumor's characteristic angiocentric growth pattern, forming structures which resembled the perivascular pseudorosettes of an ependymoma. They also observed that the tumors appeared to be biologically indolent.

Lellouch-Tubiana and coworkers described ten children who also had intractable partial seizures [2]. They similarly observed an angiocentric polarity of the tumor with glial fibrillary acidic protein (GFAP) positive, fusiform and bipolar astrocytes arranged around blood vessels. They coined the term angiocentric neuroepithelial tumor for the entity.

This chapter will review the clinical and pathologic features of these rare low grade neoplasms.

Clinical Features

Overall, angiocentric gliomas are rare neoplasms; the precise incidence of the tumor is not known. The majority of cases, as previously mentioned, are discovered in children and young adults, with a mean age of 16 years and over half of patients present in the first decade of life [3]. The tumor does not appear to have a gender predilection.

These tumors have been reported to arise in superficial cerebrocortical locations, preferentially in the frontal, parietal and temporal lobes [1, 2, 4]. Rare cases have been documented to arise in other locations, such as the brainstem [5, 6].

The majority of patients present with pharmacoresistant epilepsy, necessitating surgical intervention. Other symptoms have been less frequently encountered and have included headaches and visual disturbances [7, 8], progressive hand weakness [9], hemiparetic gait and facial nerve palsy [6], double vision and nausea [6], and psychotic symptoms [10]; these less common presentations are usually encountered in tumors arising in more unusual places.

On imaging studies, angiocentric gliomas appear to be primarily localized to superficial cortical locations but can extend to involve subcortical white matter. The tumor tends to have an infiltrative growth pattern and may, similar to other infiltrative low grade gliomas, grossly result in a blurring of the gray-white matter interface. The tumor may appear relatively circumscribed, solid, hyperintense and noncontrast enhancing on magnetic resonance imaging (MRI) FLAIR images [4, 11]. In some cases on T1-weighted MRI studies, a cortical band of hyperintensity can be seen and in other cases, a stalk-like extension of the tumor toward the subjacent lateral ventricle may be evident [2, 4, 12]. The tumors general show no appreciable mass effect.

Pathologic Features

Angiocentric gliomas are marked by a relatively monomorphic proliferation of spindled, bipolar appearing cells which have a proclivity for arranging themselves around blood vessels forming perivascular pseudorosette-like structures (Figures 1 and 2). The cells may be arranged either radially or longitudinally around the vessels. Either individual cells or multiple layers of cells may be arranged around the vessels.

In contrast to diffuse astrocytomas, satellitosis of tumor cells around neurons is not a frequent feature. Area of the tumor may show no pseudorosettes and resemble the appearance of an infiltrative diffuse astrocytoma (Figure 3). Also similar to diffuse astrocytomas, the interface between the tumor and adjacent brain parenchyma may not be clear or distinct (Figure 4). Subpial aggregation of tumor cells may be seen in some cases. Cytologically, the tumor cells are fairly monomorphic in appearance with rounded to elongated nuclei, a finely granular nuclear chromatin pattern and inconspicuous nucleoli. Cytoplasm may be scant, especially in the more spindled cells, to more prominent and eosinophilic in the more rounded or epithelioid appearing cells. Occasionally, tumors may show microcystic changes and calcification. Prominent mitotic activity is usually not present, although rare instances of tumors with increased mitotic figures (as many as 11 mitotic figures in 50 high power fields) have been documented [1]. Necrosis and vascular proliferative changes as seen in high grade gliomas are not typical features of angiocentric glioma. Rare cases of tumors with mixed features of angiocentric glioma and ependymoma have been described and rare cases of such tumors with anaplastic features have also been reported [1, 13, 14].

Similar to other low grade neoplasms associated with medically intractable epilepsy, the brain parenchyma adjacent to angiocentric gliomas may show a disorganized cortical architecture (focal cortical dysplasia) (Figure 5) [7, 15, 16]. In series of 5 angiocentric gliomas, four were noted to have focal cortical dysplasia, usually resembling the pathology described as part of an International League Against Epilepsy (ILAE) type I lesion [17]; however, because of the coexistence of the focal cortical dysplasia with a tumor, the lesion is classified as ILAE type IIIb. In one report of three tumors with coexistent focal cortical dysplasia, the pathology of the focal cortical dysplasia in one of the three cases resembled that of an ILAE type IIb lesion, marked by dysmorphic neurons and balloon cells [15]. The epilepsy in many of the focal cortical dysplasia associated tumors generally originates not from the tumor but from the adjacent architecturally disorganized cortex.

The Clinical and Pathologic Features of Angiocentric Glioma   49

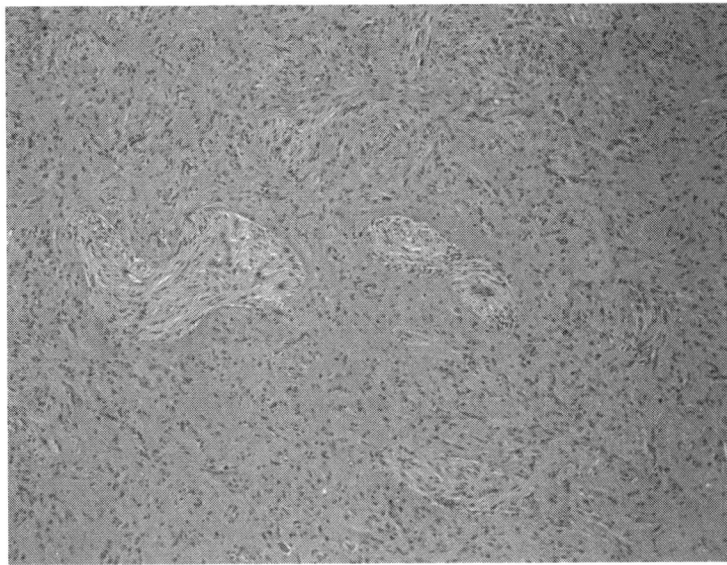

Figure 1. Low magnification appearance of an angiocentric glioma showing a mildly hypercellular neoplasm with focally spindled cells arranged around blood vessels (hematoxylin and eosin, original magnification 200X).

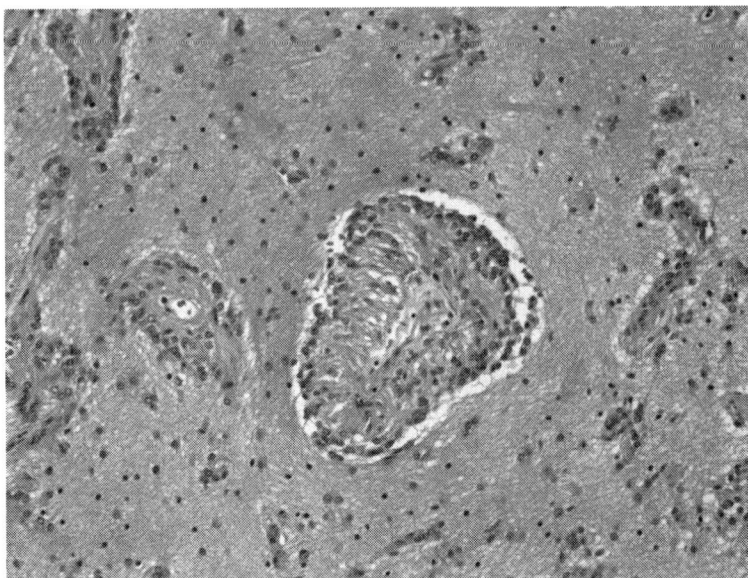

Figure 2. The characteristic angoiocentric arrangement of tumor cells around blood vessels. These cells have a slightly more epithelioid appearance (hematoxylin and eosin, original magnification 200X).

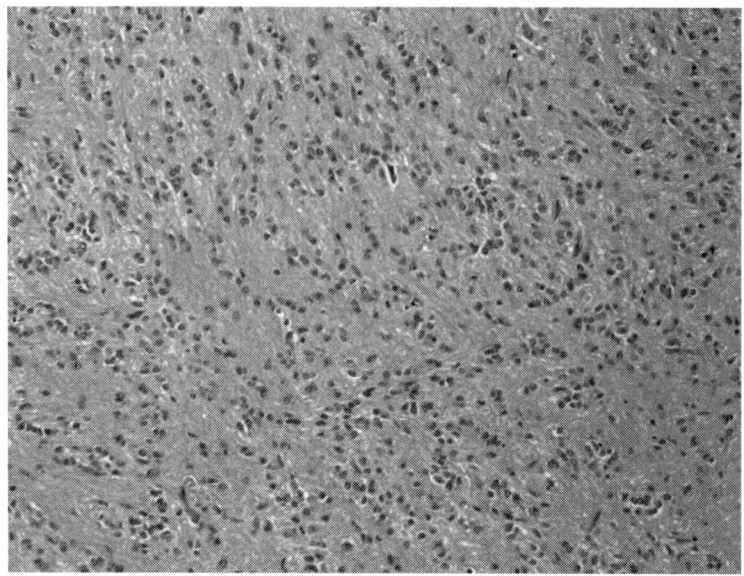

Figure 3. Focal areas of angiocentric glioma may show infiltration of brain parenchyma, resembling a diffuse astrocytoma (hematoxylin and eosin, original magnification 200X).

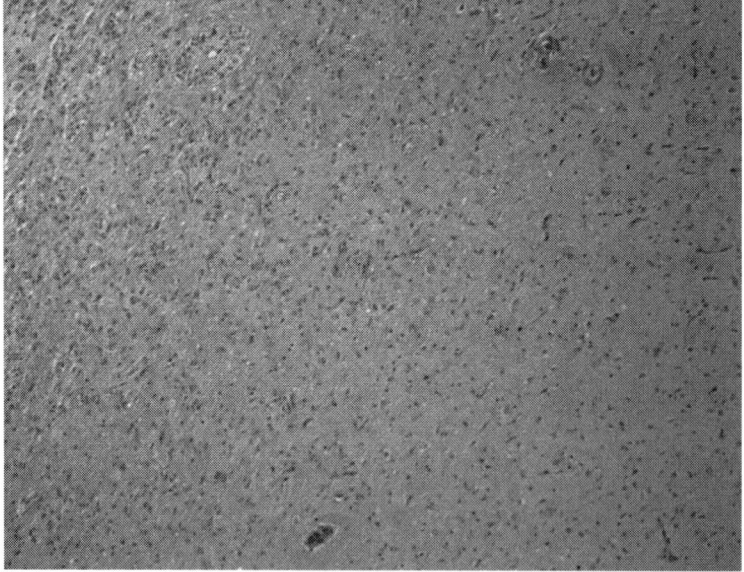

Figure 4. The interface between the tumor (left) and the adjacent uninvolved brain parenchyma (right) is not clear due to the infiltrative growth pattern of angiocentric glioma (hematoxylin and eosin, original magnification 50X).

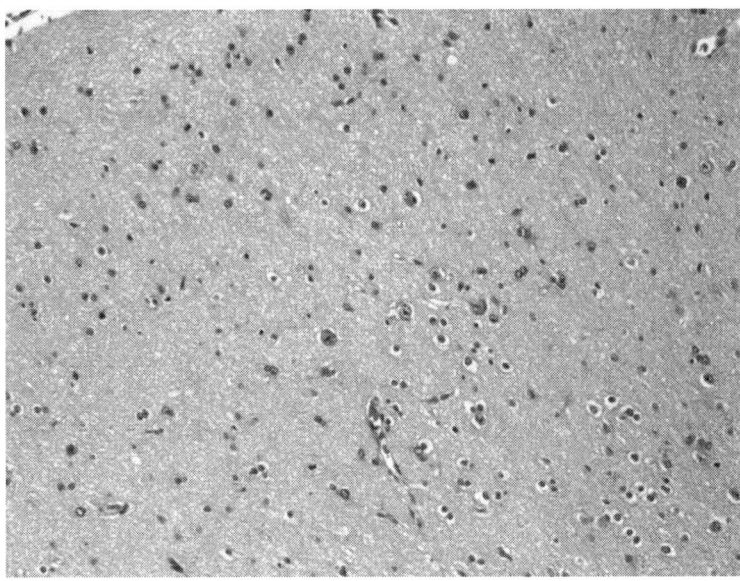

Figure 5. An area of cortical architectural disorganization or focal cortical dysplasia near an angiocentric glioma. This area of superficial cortex is marked by a loss of cortical layer II and a malpositioning of larger pyramidal neurons where layer II would normally reside (hematoxylin and eosin, original magnification 200X).

Angiocentric gliomas stain with many of the antibody stains that typically target astrocytic tumors, such as glial fibrillary acidic protein (GFAP), S-100 protein and vimentin [4]. They may show dot-like cytoplasmic staining with epithelial membrane antigen (EMA), similar to what is observed in ependymal tumors [1, 4]. Other markers of ependymal tumors such as CD99 and D2-40 may variably stain angiocentric glioma [4]. Markers of neural differentiation, such as NeuN, synaptophysin and chromogranin are not seen in these tumors [4]. Many immunomarkers that may show positive results in other low grade astrocytic neoplasms, including IDH-1 (R132H), p53 and BRAF V600E do not stain angiocentric glioma.

Cell proliferation labeling indices are typically low in angiocentric gliomas. Ki-67 or MIB-1 labeling indices are usually in the 1% to 5% range [1, 4, 7]. Only rare cases with elevated indices in the 8-10% range have been noted [1, 17-19]. The clinical significance of these elevated indices in these cases is uncertain but may be indicative of an increased likelihood of recurrence in a shorter interval of time.

As previously indicated, angiocentric gliomas do not demonstrate the IDH-1 or IDH-2, ATRX, p53 or BRAF V600E mutations encountered in other low grade gliomas [20-22]. Recent work has uncovered a genetic alteration that appears to be somewhat specific for angiocentric glioma. In 2016, Bandopadhayay and colleagues examined 19 angiocentric gliomas and noted that all of them had gene fusions that involved the MYB locus and almost all the tumors were found to have a MYB-QKI fusions [23]. In another study published in the same year, evidence of MYB-QKI fusions were found in 13 of 15 angiocentric gliomas examined [24]. Only rare chromosomal abnormalities were noted in an examination of eight tumors utilizing comparative genomic hybridization (one tumor with a gain on chromosome 11p11.2 and one tumor with a loss of chromosome 6q24-35) [4].

Electron microscopic examination of angiocentric gliomas have shown cells marked by intermediate molecular weight cytoplasmic filaments and basement membranes that are situated proximal to blood vessels [1, 4]. Studies have also noted that intercellular lumens with microvilli and cell junctions are present [1, 4]. Cilia are not present. It has been postulated that the tumors arise from bipolar radial glia and may share traits with ependymoglial cells or are capable of ependymocytic differentiation [2].

Differential Diagnoses

There are three main lesions in the differential diagnosis of angiocentric glioma. Ultrastructural and immunohistochemical findings along with the pseudorosette formations conjure up ependymoma in the differential. Ependymomas are typically intraventricular and not parenchymal based masses. They are usually circumscribed. Angiocentric gliomas also lack the formation of true rosettes, which characterize a subset of ependymomas.

Diffuse astrocytomas are also in the differential of angiocentric gliomas. Similar to angiocentric gliomas, diffuse astrocytomas are infiltrative, parenchymal based tumors. Arrangement of tumor cells around vessels may be evident in a subset of these neoplasms (so called secondary structures of Sherer); however as previously mentioned, perineuronal satellitosis is usually not a feature of angiocentric gliomas. Diffuse astrocytomas often demonstrate more nuclear pleomorphism and more commonly, especially with higher grade tumors, demonstrate more readily identifiable mitotic activity, vascular proliferation or necrosis. Immunomarkers that in a subset of diffuse astrocytomas may yield positive results (i.e., IDH-1, p53, ATRX) do not yield positive results in angiocentric gliomas.

Pilocytic astrocytomas and pilomyxoid astrocytomas may at times show an angiocentric arrangement of tumor cells. Features typical of these tumors such as Rosenthal fibers, eosinophilic granular bodies, cyst with mural nodule appearance on imaging, and BRAF abnormalities are not features of angiocentric glioma.

Treatment and Prognosis

The majority of angiocentric gliomas appear to be indolent and are probably curable with complete surgical resection. The trick, because of the infiltrative nature, is trying to know whether one has excised the entire tumor; incompletely excised tumors can grow back. They are considered grade I tumors in the World Health Organization (WHO) classification of central nervous system tumors [25]. Rare cases of recurrent tumors with anaplastic features have been documented [1, 13]. There are no features that are known to be predicative of which tumors may undergo anaplastic transformation. There is no role for adjuvant chemotherapy or radiation therapy for these tumors.

REFERENCES

[1] Wang M, Tihan T, Rojiani A, et al. Monomorphous angiocentric glioma: A distinctive epileptogenic neoplasm with features of infiltrating astrocytoma and ependymoma. *J. Neuropathol. Exp. Neurol.* 2005; 64(10): 875-881.

[2] Lellouch-Tubiana A, Boddaert N, Bourgeois M, et al. Angiocentric neuroepithelial tumor (ANET): a new epilepsy-related clinicopathological entity with distinctive MRI. *Brain Pathol.* 2005; 15(4): 281-286.

[3] Brat D J, Perry A. Other glial neoplasms. In: Perry A, Brat DJ editors. *Practical Surgical Neuropathology. A Diagnostic Approach.* 2nd Edition. Elsevier. Philadelphia, PA. 2018. pp. 171-175.

[4] Preusser M, Hoischen A, Novak K, et al. Angiocentric glioma. Report of clinico-pathologic and genetic findings in 8 cases. *Am. J. Surg. Pathol.* 2007; 31(11): 1709-1718.

[5] Covington D B, Rosenblum M K, Brathwaite C D, et al. Angiocentric glioma-like tumor of the midbrain. *Pediatr. Neurosurg.* 2009; 45: 429-433.

[6] Weaver K J, Crawford L M, Bennett J A, et al. Brainstem angiocentric glioma: report of 2 cases. *J. Neurosurg. Pediatr.* 2017; 20: 347-351.

[7] Marburger T, Prayson R. Angiocentric glioma. A clinicopathologic review of 5 tumors with identification of associated cortical dysplasia. *Arch. Pathol. Lab. Med.* 2011; 135: 1037-1041. 10.

[8] Shakur S F, McGirt M J, Johnson M W, et al. Angiocentric glioma: a case series. *J. Neurosurg. Pediatr.* 2009; 3(3): 197-202.

[9] Gonzalez-Quarante L H, Carballai C F, Agarwal V, et al. Angiocentric glioma in an elderly patient: Case report and review of the literature. *World Neursurg.* 2017; 97: 755.E5-755.E10.

[10] Kadak M T, Demirel A, Demir T. Angiocentric glioma manifesting as psychotic symptoms in an adolescent: A case report. *Neurol. Psych. Brain Res.* 2013; 19: 197-200.

[11] Burger P C, Juvet A, Presusser M, et al. Angiocentric glioma. In: Louis D N, Ohgaki H, Wiestler O D, Cavenee W K editors. *WHO Classification of Tumours of the Central Nervous System*, 4th edition. IARC Press. Lyon, FR: 2007. pp. 92-93.

[12] Koral K, Koral K M, Sklar F. Angiocentric glioma in a 4-year-old boy; imaging characteristics and review of the literature. *Clin. Imaging* 2012; 36(1): 61-64.

[13] McCracken J A, Gonzales M F, Phal P M, et al. Angiocentric glioma transformed into anaplastic ependymoma: Review of the evidence for malignant potential. *J. Clin. Neurosci.* 2016; 34: 47-52.

[14] Hiniker A, Lee H S, Chang S, et al. Cortical ependymoma with unusual histologic features. *Clin. Neuropathol.* 2013; 32(4): 318-323.

[15] Liu C Q, Zhou J, Qi X L, et al. Refractory temporal lobe epilepsy caused by angiocentric glioma complicated with focal cortical dysplasia: a surgical case series. *J. Neurooncol.* 2012; 110: 375-380.

[16] Takeda S, Iwasaki M, Suzuki H, et al. Angiocentric glioma and surrounding cortical dysplasia manifesting as intractable frontal epilepsy. Case report. *Neurol Med Chir (Tokyo)* 2011; 51: 522-526.

[17] Pokharel S, Parker J R, Parker J C, et al. Angiocentric glioma with high proliferative index: Case report and review of the literature. *Ann. Clin. Lab. Sci.* 2011; 41(3): 257-261.

[18] Sugita Y, Ono T, Ohshima K, et al. Brain surface spindle cell glioma in a patient with medically intractable partial epilepsy: A variant of monomorphous angiocentric glioma? *Neuropathology* 2008; 28: 516-520.

[19] Li J, Adesina A, Bodhireddy S R, et al. Angiocentric glioma: Elevated proliferation rate at clinical presentation does not preclude extended recurrence-free survival. *FASEB J.* 2008; 22: 706.6.

[20] Raghunathan A, Olar A, Vogel H, et al. Isocitrate dehydrogenase 1 R132H mutation is not detected in angiocentric glioma. *Ann. Diagn. Pathol.* 2012; 16: 255-259.

[21] Ni H-C, Chen S-Y, Chen L, et al. Angiocentric gliomas: a report of nine new cases, including four with atypical histological features. *Neuropathol. Appl. Neurobiol.* 2014; 41(3): 333-346.

[22] Buccoliero A M, Castiglione F, Degl'innocenti D R, et al. Angiocentric glioma: clinical, morphological, immunohistochemical and molecular features in three pediatric cases. *Clin. Neuropathol.* 2013; 32(2): 107-113.

[23] Bandopadhayay P, Ramkissooon L A, Resnick A C. MYB-QKI rearrangements in angiocentric glioma drive tumorigenicity through a tripartite mechanism. *Nature Genet.* 2016; 48: 273-282.

[24] Qaddoumi I, Orisme W, Wen J, et al. Genetic alterations in uncommon low-grade neuroepithelial tumors: BRAF, FGFR1, and MYB mutations occur at high frequency and align with morphology. *Acta. Neuropathol.* 2016; 131(6): 833-845.

[25] Burger P C, Jouvet A, Preusser M, et al. Angiocentric glioma. In: Louis DN, Ohgaki H, Wiestler OD, Cavenee WK, eds. *WHO Classification of Tumours of the Central Nervous System.* IARC Press. Lyon, FR. 2016. pp. 119-120.

In: Tumors of the Central Nervous System
Editor: James A. Reed
ISBN: 978-1-53619-628-3
© 2021 Nova Science Publishers, Inc.

Chapter 5

CHORDOID GLIOMAS: PATHOLOGICAL AND CLINICAL ASPECTS

Anas M. Saad, MD and Richard A. Prayson, MD, MEd*
Department of Anatomic Pathology,
Cleveland Clinic, Cleveland, OH, US

ABSTRACT

Chordoid gliomas (CG) are rare neoplasms of the central nervous system that arise from the roof or the anterior wall of the third ventricle and are more common in middle-aged females. CG are non-invasive and can be asymptomatic or present with non-specific neurological symptoms that vary depending on size and location of the tumor. On magnetic resonance imaging (MRI), CG appear as a well-circumscribed tumor with a round or an oval shape. Chordoid glioma was first described in 1995 and was later classified as a grade II neoplasm by the World Health Organization (WHO). Morphologically, the tumor is marked by a proliferation of cohesive clusters of epithelioid cells with prominent eosinophilic cytoplasm and a vacuolated appearing, mucin-rich stroma. The tumor is typically accompanied by a lymphoplasmacytic infiltrate with Russell bodies. CG stain with antibodies to glial fibrillary acidic

---

* Corresponding Author's E-mail: praysor@ccf.org.

protein (GFAP), CD34, and thyroid transcription factor 1 (TTF-1). It has been variously hypothesized that CG originate from glial ependymal cells or from the organum vasculosum. Tumor-directed surgery is the mainstay of treatment of GC. Most tumors do well clinically upon gross total resection; however, cases will recur if not completely resected and can cause complications and death related to tumor location. In this chapter, we will review the histological and clinical features of chordoid gliomas.

INTRODUCTION

Chordoid gliomas (CG) are rare neoplasms (with less than 100 cases described in the literature [1]) that arise from the central nervous system (CNS) and they are hypothesized to originate from ependymal cells. It was first described in 1995 as a variant of meningioma [2]. Later, it was reported as a distinct entity in 1998 in a case series of 8 patients [3], before being included as a distinct and separate clinicopathologic entity in the 2000 (and then 2007 and 2016) World Health Organization classification of brain tumors, as a grade II glioma [4–6]. CGs are more likely to arise in females with a ratio of 2:1 [1], and occur predominantly in middle-aged individuals, with a median age of 48 years [7], although there are a few reported cases in children as young as 5 or 13 years [7, 8]. In this chapter, we will review the histological and clinical features of chordoid gliomas.

ETIOLOGY

The origin of chordoid gliomas are still not completely understood. One hypothesis suggests that GC may raise from ependymal cells [9, 10], which is supported by the expression of CD99 [10]. Four previous cases were reported where GC were associated with a different histological component; Rathke's cleft cyst in 1 case [11], epidermoid cyst in 1 case [12], and Rosai-Dorfman disease in 2 cases [13]. Despite the increase of reported cases of GC, the exact etiology remains unclear and requires further study.

CLINICAL PRESENTATION

Most cases of CG arise from the anterior wall of the third ventricle. However, there have been some reported cases of CG arising in other locations, including the lateral ventricle [14], the fourth ventricle [15], the thalamus [16], and cerebellar hemispheres [1, 14].

CG are generally benign, slow-growing, and non-invasive, with a wide variety of symptoms correlated with the tumor location, including headache, cognitive changes and memory problems, visual field defects, visual acuity decline, drowsiness, nausea, vomiting, endocrine abnormalities, hypothalamic dysfunction, neurogenic fever and other symptoms [17–19]. Similarly, the onset of symptoms differs significantly between patients based on the size and location of the tumor [18]. Incidental presentation of CG is relatively uncommon with very few patients reported to have presented asymptomatically [7]. Some reports have indicated invasion of the optic structures [20]. One case reported post-surgical recurrence with rapid progression, leading to a poor prognosis and death in less than a year following diagnosis [21]. Despite its low grade and its generally benign course, CG can be associated with severe morbidity and poor prognosis, if located in vital parts of the brain.

IMAGING

On enhanced magnetic resonance imaging (MRI), CG appears as a well-circumscribed lesion with an oval or round shape. It shows mild hyperintensity on T2-weighted images, while being isointense on T1-weighted images [22]. Following gadolinium injection, CG appear to have strong homogenous enhancement, with cystic changes and necrosis found in a few cases [22]. Some rare cases have reported the presence of calcification on both imaging and gross examination [23]. Unfortunately, imaging cannot confirm the diagnosis, and the differential diagnoses include other brain tumors that might arise in this region like meningiomas, craniopharyngiomas, and others [24]. The presence of perifocal edema is helps in making the diagnosis of CG. Patient characteristics and clinical presentation are also crucial in making the diagnosis and can help exclude other possible diagnoses [23, 24]. The presence of a dural extension or "tail" suggests a meningioma. However, due to its similar location and its prevalence among similar population groups, craniopharyngioma is generally harder to distinguish. Many craniopharyngiomas demonstrate calcifications but this is not very specific, given the reporting of calcification in some CG cases [23].

HISTOPATHOLOGY

Under the microscope, CG usually show clusters and cords of eosinophilic epithelioid tumor cells within a variably vacuolated appearing mucinous stroma (Figure 1) that typically contains a lymphocytic and plasma cell infiltrate (Figure 2), occasionally showing Russell bodies (Figure 3). Tumor cells are fairly monomorphic with generally rounded nuclei and occasional small nucleoli and eosinophilic cytoplasm, with few mitotic figures and generally no necrosis or vascular proliferation (Figure 4). Occasionally, tumor cells may assume a more spindled appearance (Figure 5) [1].

In addition, CG have been reported to stain with antibodies to glial fibrillary acidic protein (GFAP), microtubule-associated protein 2 (MAP2), S-100 protein, epithelial membrane antigen (EMA), epithelial growth factor receptor (EGFR), schwannomin, vimentin, CD34, and thyroid transcription factor 1 (TTF-1), the last two being considered the most useful [1, 24–28]. Some cases also reported synaptophysin, CD31, and E-cadherin expression [9, 29]. Most published cases, with only few exceptions, report a Ki-67 proliferation index that is less than 5% [1, 28].

Using comparative genomic hybridization, a study reported no chromosomal imbalances, TP53 and CKN2A aberrations, or EGFR, CKD4, and MDM2 amplifications [28].

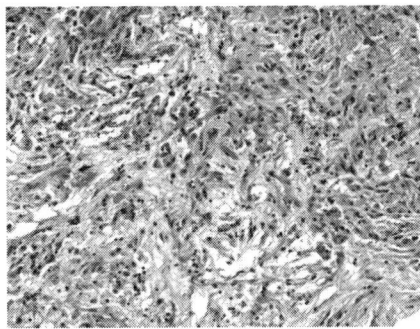

Figure 1. Clusters of epithelioid cells arranged against a mucin-rich background is characteristic of chordoid glioma (hematoxylin and eosin, original magnification 200X).

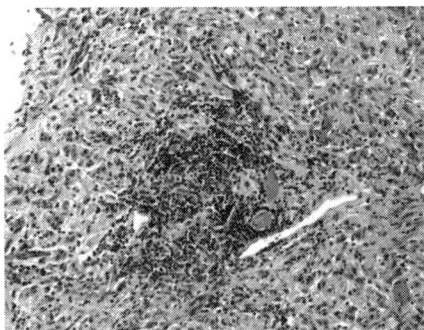

Figure 2. Collections of lymphocytes and plasma cells are commonly encountered in chordoid gliomas (hematoxylin and eosin, original magnification 200X).

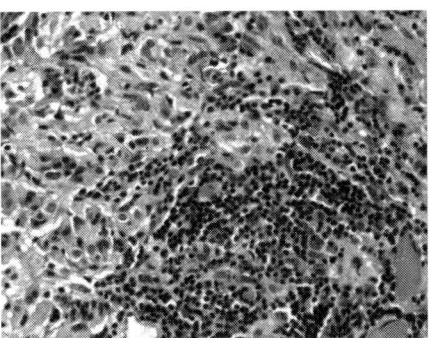

Figure 3. Small rounded eosinophilic structures, Russell bodies, are also a common feature of the chordoid glioma (hematoxylin and eosin, original magnification 400X).

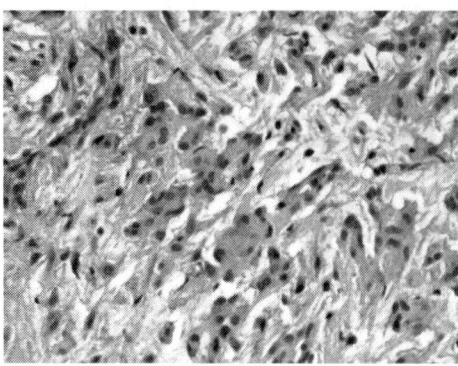

Figure 4. Tumor cells are fairly monomorphic with generally rounded nuclei and occasional small nucleoli and eosinophilic cytoplasm (hematoxylin and eosin, original magnification 400X).

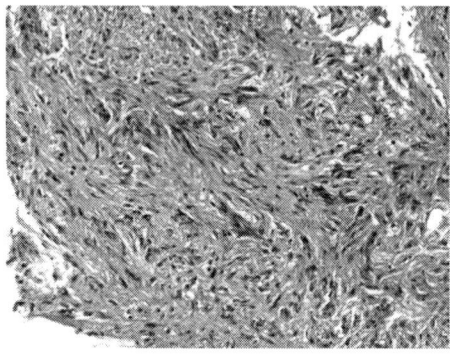

Figure 5. Occasionally, tumor cells may acquire a more spindled appearance (hematoxylin and eosin, original magnification 200X).

Another study, using fluorescence in situ hybridization showed consistent 9p21 and 11q13 alterations [29]. More recent genomic profiling studies have identified recurrent mutations in the PRKCA gene in most studied cases, with few cases also showing $BRAF^{V600E}$ mutations [27, 30].

Pathologic differential diagnoses include pituitary adenoma, meningioma and chordoma. Pituitary adenomas are typically marked by a more epithelioid appearance and usually lack the mucinous matrix and lymphoplasmacytic infiltrate typical of chordoid gliomas. They often stain with synaptophysin and pituitary hormone stains. Meningiomas may focally have a chordoid appearance which might resemble a chordoid glioma. Typical meningiomas stain with markers for epithelial membrane antigen, progesterone receptor and somatostatin receptor 2a (SSTR2a). The whorling pattern of meningioma and psammoma bodies are other meningioma features that are not typical of a chordoid glioma. Chordomas are usually located in the clivus region but may occasionally be seen in the hypothalamic region. The physaliferous or bubble-like cytoplasm which marks chordoma cells is not a feature of chordoid glioma.

MANAGEMENT

Given its rarity, no clear guidelines exist for the management and treatment of CG. Gross total resection is the most common treatment for these patients, with the most common approaches including transcallosal, transcortical, and trans-lamina terminalis; the last is associated with the lowest risks of post-operative complications [7]. However, surgical resection is relatively challenging (and sometimes not possible) because of the tumor's location, [1] and post-operative mortality rates can be as high as 17%, with most deaths being attributed to infections or pulmonary embolism [23]. Tumors proximal to the hypothalamus are specifically challenging and are associated with higher risk of post-operative hypothalamic dysfunction and syndrome of inappropriate antidiuretic hormone [7]. Other reported post-operative complications include panhypopituitarism, new-onset seizures, short-term memory problems, personality changes, hyperphagia and weight gain, hematoma, pneumonia, bacterial meningitis, pulmonary embolism, and electrolyte disturbances [7, 17]. On the other hand, partial resection can be performed in some cases, but it has been found to be associated with high recurrence rates [31]. Progression-free survival after 5 years of partial resection is estimated to be only about 35.5% [32].

Some have suggested the use of radiosurgery, or radiotherapy following resection, but this has been associated with variable results, and with recurrence still remaining an important concern [33, 34]. On the other hand, no published cases, to our knowledge, report the use of chemotherapy.

Following treatment, and despite the relatively high short term morbidity and mortality rates, the conditional cause-specific survival of patients who recover following surgery is generally favorable [17].

REFERENCES

[1] Zhang G Bin, Huang HW, Li HY, et al. Intracranial chordoid glioma: A clinical, radiological and pathological study of 14 cases. *J. Clin. Neurosci.* [Internet]. 2020;80:267–273. Available from: https://doi.org/10.1016/j.jocn.2020.09.019.

[2] Wanschitz J, Schmidbauer M, Maier H, et al. Suprasellar meningioma with expression of glial fibrillary acidic protein: a peculiar variant. *Acta Neuropathol.* [Internet]. 1995;90:539–544. Available from: http://link.springer.com/10.1007/BF00294817.

[3] Brat DJ, Scheithauer BW, Staugaitis SM, et al. Third ventricular chordoid glioma: A distinct clinicopathologic entity. *J. Neuropathol. Exp. Neurol.* [Internet]. 1998;57:283–290. Available from: https://academic.oup.com/jnen/article-lookup/doi/10.1097/00005072-199803000-00009.

[4] Louis DN, Ohgaki H, Wiestler OD, et al. The 2007 WHO classification of tumours of the central nervous system. *Acta Neuropathol.* 2007;114:97–109.

[5] Louis DN, Perry A, Reifenberger G, et al. The 2016 World Health Organization Classification of Tumors of the Central Nervous System: a summary. *Acta Neuropathol.* 2016;131:803–820.

[6] Gonzales M. The 2000 World Health Organization classification of tumours of the nervous system. *J. Clin. Neurosci.* [Internet]. 2001;8:1–3. Available from: https://linkinghub.elsevier.com/retrieve/pii/S0967586800908294.

[7] Ampie L, Choy W, Lamano JB, et al. Prognostic factors for recurrence and complications in the surgical management of primary

chordoid gliomas: A systematic review of literature. *Clin. Neurol. Neurosurg.* [Internet]. 2015;138:129–136. Available from: https://linkinghub.elsevier.com/retrieve/pii/S0303846715002875.

[8] Morais BA, Menendez DFS, Medeiros RSS, et al. Chordoid glioma: Case report and review of the literature. *Int. J. Surg. Case Rep.* [Internet]. 2015;7:168–171. Available from: http://dx.doi.org/10.1016/j.ijscr.2015.01.027.

[9] Sato K, Kubota T, Ishida M, et al. Immunohistochemical and ultrastructural study of chordoid glioma of the third ventricle: its tanycytic differentiation. *Acta Neuropathol.* [Internet]. 2003;106:176–180. Available from: http://link.springer.com/10.1007/s00401-003-0713-2.

[10] Romero-Rojas AE, Díaz-Pérez JA, Ariza-Serrano LM. CD99 is expressed in chordoid glioma and suggests ependymal origin. *Virchows Arch.* 2012;460:119–122.

[11] Suh Y-L, Kim NR, Kim J-H, et al. Suprasellar chordoid glioma combined with Rathke's cleft cyst. *Pathol. Int.* [Internet]. 2003;53:780–785. Available from: http://doi.wiley.com/10.1046/j.1440-1827.2003.01549.x.

[12] Poyuran R, Mahadevan A, Sagar BKC, et al. Chordoid glioma of third ventricle with an epidermoid cyst. *Int. J. Surg. Pathol.* [Internet]. 2016;24:663–667. Available from: http://journals.sagepub.com/doi/10.1177/1066896916650256.

[13] Yao K, Duan Z, Ma Z, et al. Concurrence of chordoid gliomas with Rosai-Dorfman component: Report of two rare cases. *Int. J. Clin. Exp. Pathol.* 2017;10:11260–11266.

[14] Yang B, Yang C, Du J, et al. Chordoid glioma: an entity occurring not exclusively in the third ventricle. *Neurosurg. Rev.* 2020;43:1315–1322.

[15] Lee YS, Yeung TW, Leung OC. One of a kind—chordoid glioma in the fourth ventricle: a case report and literature review. *Acta Radiol. Open.* 2020;9:205846012098014.

[16] Kim JW, Kim JH, Choe G, et al. Chordoid glioma : A case report of unusual location and neuroradiological characteristics. *J. Korean*

Neurosurg. Soc. [Internet]. 2010;48:62. Available from: http://jkns.or.kr/journal/view.php?doi=10.3340/jkns.2010.48.1.62.

[17] Huo CW, Rathi V, Scarlett A, et al. The trans-laminar terminalis approach reduces mortalities associated with chordoid glioma resections: A case report and a review of 20 years of literature. *J. Clin. Neurosci.* [Internet]. 2018;47:43–55. Available from: https://doi.org/10.1016/j.jocn.2017.10.029.

[18] Calanchini M, Cudlip S, Hofer M, et al. Chordoid glioma of the third ventricle: a patient presenting with SIADH and a review of this rare tumor. *Pituitary.* 2016;19:356–361.

[19] García Carretero R, Romero Brugera M, Vazquez-Gomez O, et al. Neurogenic fever in a patient with a chordoid glioma. *BMJ Case Rep.* 2016;2016:1–4.

[20] Sanda N, Mircea CN, Bernier M, et al. Chordoid glioma infiltrating optic structures. *J. Neuroophthalmol.* 2019;39:408–410.

[21] Erwood AA, Velazquez-Vega JE, Neill S, et al. Chordoid glioma of the third ventricle: report of a rapidly progressive case. *J. Neurooncol.* 2017;132:487–495.

[22] Qixing F, Peiyi G, Kai W, et al. The radiological findings of chordoid glioma: report of two cases, one case with MR spectroscopy. *Clin. Imaging* [Internet]. 2015;39:1086–1089. Available from: https://linkinghub.elsevier.com/retrieve/pii/S0899707115001709.

[23] Cui Z, Mu C, Yang F, et al. A rare instance of chordoid glioma with large calcification mimicking craniopharyngioma. *J. Craniofac. Surg.* 2020;31:e173–e175.

[24] Shinohara T, Inoue A, Kohno S, et al. Usefulness of neuroimaging and immunohistochemical study for accurate diagnosis of chordoid glioma of the third ventricle: A case report and review of the literature. *Surg. Neurol. Int.* [Internet]. 2018;9:226. Available from: http://surgicalneurologyint.com/surgicalint-articles/usefulness-of-neuroimaging-and-immunohistochemical-study-for-accurate-diagnosis-of-chordoid-glioma-of-the-third-ventricle-a-case-report-and-review-of-the-literature/.

[25] Michotte A, Van Der Veken J, Huylebrouck M, et al. Expression of thyroid transcription factor 1 in a chordoid glioma. *J. Neurol. Sci.* [Internet]. 2014;346:362–363. Available from: http://dx.doi.org/10.1016/j.jns.2014.09.005.

[26] Hewer E, Beck J, Kellner-Weldon F, et al. Suprasellar chordoid neoplasm with expression of thyroid transcription factor 1: Evidence that chordoid glioma of the third ventricle and pituicytoma may form part of a spectrum of lineage-related tumors of the basal forebrain. *Hum. Pathol.* [Internet]. 2015;46:1045–1049. Available from: http://dx.doi.org/10.1016/j.humpath.2015.03.005.

[27] Yao K, Duan Z, Du Z, et al. PRKCA D463H mutation in chordoid glioma of the third ventricle: A cohort of 16 cases, including two cases harboring BRAFV600E mutation. *J. Neuropathol. Exp. Neurol.* 2020;79:1183–1192.

[28] Reifenberger G, Weber T, Weber RG, et al. Chordoid glioma of the third ventricle: immunohistochemical and molecular genetic characterization of a novel tumor entity. *Brain Pathol.* [Internet]. 1999;9:617–626. Available from: http://doi.wiley.com/10.1111/j.1750-3639.1999.tb00543.x.

[29] Horbinski C, Dacic S, McLendon RE, et al. Chordoid glioma: A case report and molecular characterization of five cases. *Brain Pathol.* [Internet]. 2009;19:439–448. Available from: http://doi.wiley.com/10.1111/j.1750-3639.2008.00196.x.

[30] Goode B, Mondal G, Hyun M, et al. A recurrent kinase domain mutation in PRKCA defines chordoid glioma of the third ventricle. *Nat. Commun.* 2018;9.

[31] Yang D, Xu Z, Qian Z, et al. Chordoid glioma: A neoplasm found in the anterior part of the third ventricle. *J. Craniofac. Surg.* 2017;00:1–3.

[32] Destefani MH, Mello AS, Oliveira RS de, et al. Chordoid glioma of the third ventricle. *Radiol. Bras.* [Internet]. 2015;48:338–339. Available from: http://www.scielo.br/scielo.php?script=sci_arttext&pid=S0100-39842015000500338&lng=en&tlng=en.

[33] DeSouza R-M, Bodi I, Thomas N, et al. Chordoid glioma: Ten years of a low-grade tumor with high morbidity. *Skull Base* [Internet]. 2010;20:125–138. Available from: http://www.thieme-connect.de/DOI/DOI?10.1055/s-0029-1246223.

[34] Kobayashi T, Tsugawa T, Hashisume C, et al. Therapeutic approach to chordoid glioma of the third ventricle. *Neurol. Med. Chir. (Tokyo).* [Internet]. 2013;53:249–255. Available from: http://jlc.jst.go.jp/DN/JST.JSTAGE/nmc/53.249?lang=en&from=CrossRef&type=abstract.

In: Tumors of the Central Nervous System ISBN: 978-1-53619-628-3
Editor: James A. Reed © 2021 Nova Science Publishers, Inc.

Chapter 6

DYSPLASTIC GANGLIOCYTOMA OF THE CEREBELLUM (LHERMITTE-DUCLOS DISEASE): A CLINICOPATHOLOGIC REVIEW

Richard A. Prayson, MD, MEd*
Cleveland Clinic, Department of Anatomic Pathology,
Cleveland, OH, US

ABSTRACT

Dysplastic cerebellar gangliocytomas, also referred to as Lhermitte-Duclos disease, are rare low grade tumors of the cerebellar hemisphere that were first described in 1920. Most cases present in adulthood and the lesion is associated with PTEN mutations and Cowden syndrome. They typically present with signs and symptoms of mass effect, obstructive hydrocephalus and increased intracranial pressure. On imaging studies, they appear as distortions of the cerebellar hemispheric architecture with enlarged cerebellar folia and sometimes cystic changes. Histologically, they are marked by an abnormal collection of large ganglionic cells. There is no evidence of a glioma component in these lesions, such as one might see in a ganglioglioma. Mitotic activity, necrosis or vascular

---

* Corresponding Author's E-mail: praysor@ccf.org.

proliferative changes are not typically seen. The ganglion cells stain with immunomarkers typically used to highlight neuronal cells, such as synaptophysin. Surgical resection is curative in the majority of cases, but local recurrence may be encountered in a subset of cases. Patients should be followed for other manifestations of Cowden syndrome.

INTRODUCTION

The entity of dysplastic cerebellar gangliocytoma was first described slightly over 100 years ago in 1920 by Lhermitte and Duclos, hence the synonymous name Lhermitte-Duclos disease [1], and Spiegel [2]. The disease has also been referred to by a variety of other names including gangliomatosis of the cerebellum, diffuse hypertrophy of the cerebellar cortex, Purkinjeoma, granule cell hypertrophy of the cerebellum and diffuse hypertrophy of the cerebellar cortex [3]. There has been debate over whether the lesion represents an actual neoplasm or a hamartoma. Either way, it is designated by the World Health Organization (WHO) classification of brain tumors as corresponding to a grade I lesion [3].

Cowden Disease

Dysplastic cerebellar gangliocytomas are recognized as being associated with Cowden disease [4-7]. Cowden disease is an autosomal dominant disorder marked by the presence of multiple hamartomatous and neoplastic lesions of the brain, skin, colon, breast, thyroid, endometrium and mucous membrane [8]. The disease was first recognized in the early 1960s by Lloyd and Dennis [9] and is part of a spectrum of disorders marked by mutations in the phosphatase and tensin homolog (PTEN) tumor suppressor gene [10].

The protein encoded for by the PTEN gene is involved with the control of apoptosis and the cell cycle [11]. The protein product of PTEN works as a tumor suppressor via its lipid phosphatase activity and regulating the phosphatidylinositol 3-kinase pathway [12-13]. Loss of PTEN function results in an increased cell proliferation and cell survival, resulting in tumorigenesis. A variety of cancer types have somatic mutations in PTEN including breast and endometrial carcinomas and melanoma [14-16]. When heterozygosity for the PTEN gene is lost by a second hit mutation, the result is a proclivity for the development of multiple hamartomas and tumors [17].

A subset of Cowden disease patients do not have PTEN mutations but have other germline mutations in SDHB, SDHC and SDHD [18, 19]. Bennett et al. also described hypermethylation of the KILLIN promoter in some individuals with Cowden disease [20].

Criteria for the diagnosis of PTEN hamartoma tumor syndrome were adopted by the United States National Comprehensive Cancer Network in 2017 [10, 21]. Diagnosis requires that the patient have three or more major criteria with at least one of those criteria being macrocephaly, Lhermitte-Duclos disease, or gastrointestinal hamartomas. Alternatively, a patient may be diagnosed with two major and three minor criteria. In a family where one individual meets diagnostic criteria or has a PTEN mutation, then a diagnosis can be made if a patient has any two major criteria, or one major and two minor criteria or three minor criteria. The list of major criteria includes the following: breast cancer, endometrial cancer (epithelial), thyroid cancer (follicular), three or more gastrointestinal hamartomas (including ganglioneuromas but excluding hyperplastic polyps), Lhermitte-Duclos disease as an adult, macrocephaly (97th percentile or greater), macular pigmentation of the glans penis, multiple mucocutaneous lesions, three or more trichilemmomas, three or more acral keratosis lesions (palmoplantar keratotic pits or acral hyperkeratotic papules), three or more mucocutaneous neuromas, and three or more oral papillomas. Minor criteria include the following: autism spectrum disorder, colon cancer, three or more foci of esophageal glycogenic acanthosis, three or more lipomas, mental retardation (intelligence quotient of 75 or lower), renal cell carcinoma, testicular lipomatosis, thyroid cancer (papillary), thyroid structural lesions (adenoma or multinodular goiter), and vascular anomalies.

Clinical Features

Dysplastic cerebellar gangliocytomas are relatively rare lesions. They typically present during the third or fourth decades of life, although rare cases of congenital tumor have been described and rare cases may be seen in older adults up to 74 years of age [3, 22, 23]. The prevalence rate is estimated at about 1 case per million population based on a clinical epidemiologic study [24]; a molecular based estimation of the prevalence is about 1 in 200,000 individuals [25]. In a study by Riegert-Johnson and colleagues, of the 211 Cowden disease patients reviewed, 32% developed a dysplastic cerebellar gangliocytoma [26].

The most common clinical symptoms associated with presentation include seizures, ataxia or symptoms related to obstructive hydrocephalus, or increased intracranial pressure. Cranial nerve deficits have been described and rarely patients may present with orthostatic hypotension or acute subarachnoid hemorrhage. Macrocephaly is often present. The duration of symptoms prior to surgery is quite variable but in one study was determined to be on average 40 months [5]. Because of the association of this entity with Cowden disease, patients diagnosed with a cerebellar dysplastic gangliocytoma should be regularly monitored for the potential development of other cancers elsewhere in the body.

On imaging studies, the lesion typically presents as a unilateral nonenhancing cerebellar hemispheric expansion. Some cases may show cystic changes. Magnetic resonance imaging (MRI) studies often demonstrate characteristic T1-hypointense and T2-hyperintense parallel linear striations, sometimes referred to as tiger stripes. [27-29]. Perfusion imaging has shown increased relative cerebral blood volume, blood flow and mean transit time in the lesion [30].

Pathology

Grossly, the cerebellar folia in the affected area appears thickened and it appears to blend into adjacent more normal appearing folia. The enlarged folia may have a pale appearance due to an associated abnormally of myelination. The affected area may also appear firm. Occasionally, cystic changes may be evident grossly.

Histologically, the lesion often has a fairly sharp demarcation with the adjacent relatively normal cerebellar tissue (Figure 1). The mass is marked by an abnormal aggregation of hypertrophic appearing ganglion cells, often situated primarily in the internal granular cell layer (Figures 2 and 3). In some cases, the molecular layer of the cerebellum may show increased number of these atypical ganglion cells. Abnormalities of myelination, particularly in the molecular layer, are often present, resulting from the myelination of the abnormal ganglion cells that comprise the lesion. Purkinje cells are typically decreased in numbers in and near the lesion. Microcytic degeneration in and adjacent to the lesion (Figure 4), microcalcifications (Figure 5) and ectatic blood vessels may be evident. Mitotic activity, vascular proliferative changes and necrosis are not typically encountered.

Immunostains which target neuronal cells, such as neurofilament, synaptophysin, chromogranin and NeuN will highlight the ganglionic cells. Glial fibrillary acidic protein (GFAP) is typically negative in these lesions. Most of the atypical ganglion cells in the lesion do not stain with markers which target Purkinje cells (e.g., LEU4, PCP2, PCP4), which has led some to suggest that the cells in this lesion are more likely derived from internal granular cell neurons [3, 31]. Cell proliferation markers, such as Ki-67, show very low rates of cell proliferation [31, 32].

Differential Diagnosis

The major differential diagnostic consideration for the dysplastic cerebellar gangliocytoma would be a ganglioglioma. Gangliogliomas are typically circumscribed masses which are comprised of an atypical ganglionic component, similar to Lhermitte-Duclos disease, and an atypical glioma component (which is not seen in the dysplastic cerebellar gangliocytoma). The foliar enlargement growth pattern of the dysplastic cerebellar gangliocyoma would be very atypical for a ganglioglioma. Gangliogliomas often have perivascular chronic inflammation and eosinophilic granular bodies, which would be unusual in a dysplastic cerebellar gangliocytoma.

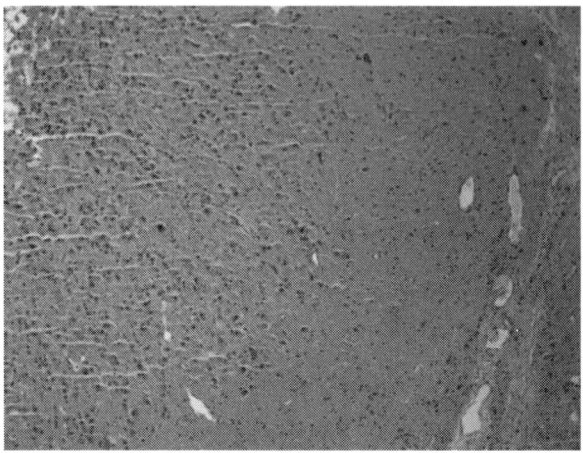

Figure 1. Dysplastic cerebellar gangliocytoma arising in the region of the internal granular cell layer and showing a fairly circumscribed interface with the adjacent uninvolved molecular layer (right) (hematoxylin and eosin, original magnification 100X).

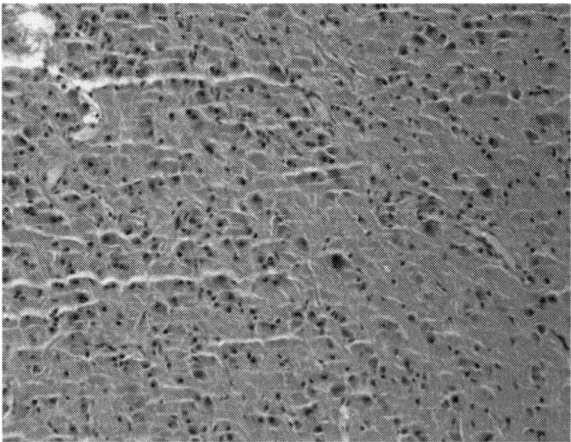

Figure 2. The tumor is comprised of an aggregation of hypertrophic ganglionic cells (hematoxylin and eosin, original magnification 200X).

Dysplastic Gangliocytoma of the Cerebellum ...   75

The genetics of ganglioglioma are also different; many show evidence of BRAF V600E mutations, which are not a feature of cerebellar dysplastic gangliocytomas.[33].

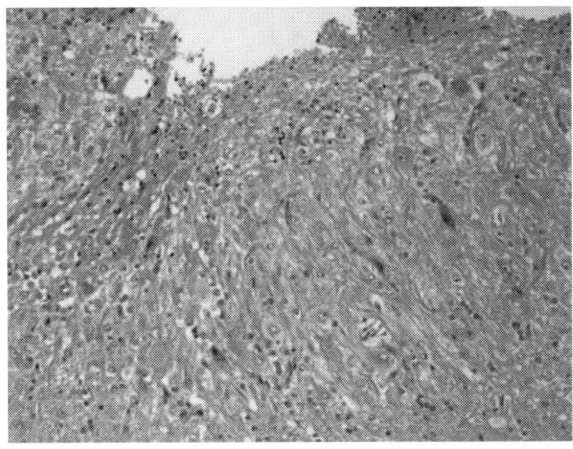

Figure 3. Large atypical ganglionic cells with a small population of intermixed granular cells with rounded nuclei (hematoxylin and eosin, original magnification 200X).

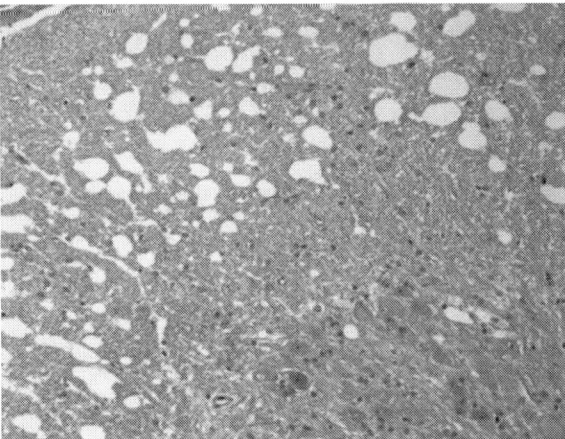

Figure 4. Microcystic changes adjacent to a dysplastic cerebellar gangliocytoma (hematoxylin and eosin, original magnification 200X).

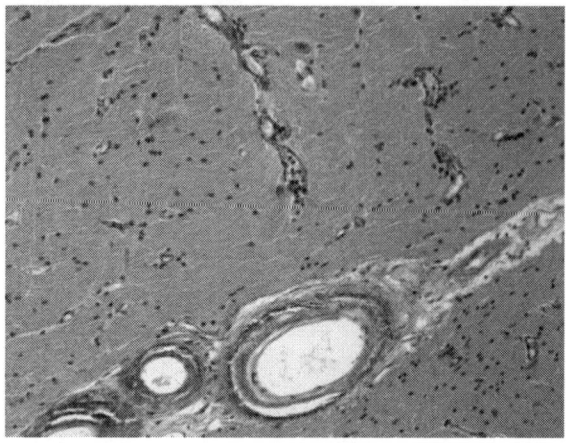

Figure 5. Microcalcifications within blood vessel walls adjacent to a dysplastic cerebellar gangliocytoma in the overlying meninges and molecular layer (hematoxylin and eosin, original magnification 200X).

TREATMENT AND PROGNOSIS

Dysplastic cerebellar gangliocytomas, as previously mentioned, are considered low grade lesions [3] which are amenable to surgical resection; surgical resection is generally considered curative. Local recurrence has been documented in a subset of cases [34]. It is debated as to whether or not recurrences suggest that the process is neoplastic or whether the recurrences may be related to hypertrophy of residual abnormal tissue [22, 34]. A diagnosis should prompt consideration of Cowden disease and careful monitoring for other malignancies associated with PTEN mutations.

REFERENCES

[1] Lhermitte J, Duclos P. Sur un ganglioneuroma diffus du coertex du cervelet. *Bull. Assoc. Fr. Etud. Cancer* 1920; 9: 99-107.

[2] Spiegel E. Hyperplasie des Kleinhims. *Bietr. Pathol. Anat.* 1920; 67: 539-548.

[3] Eberhart G, Wiestler O D, Eng C. Dysplastic cerebellar gangliocytoma (Lhermitte-Duclos disease. In: *WHO Classification of Tumours of the Central Nervous System.* Louis N, Ohgaki H, Wiestler OD, et al. (Eds). IARC Press. Lyon, FR. 2016; pp. 142-143.

[4] Eng C, Murday V, Sea l S, et al. Cowden syndrome and Lhermitte-Duclos disease in a family; a single genetic syndrome with pleiotrophy. *J. Med. Genet.* 1994; 31(6): 458-461.

[5] Vinchon M, Blond S, Lejeune J P, et al. Association of Lhermitte-Duclos and Cowden disease: report of a new case and review of the literature. *J. Neurol. Neurosurg. Psychiatry* 1994; 57(6): 699-704.

[6] Padberg G W, Schot J D, Vielvoye G J, et al. Lhermitte-Duclos disease and Cowden disease: a single phakomatosis. *Ann. Neurol.* 1991; 29(5): 517-523.

[7] Vital A, Vital C, Martin-Negrier M L, et al. Lhermitte-Duclos type cerebellum hamartoma and Cowden disease. *Clin. Neuropathol.* 1994; 13(4): 229-231.

[8] Uppal S, Mistry D, Coatesworth AP. Cowden disease: a review. *Int. J. Clin. Pract.* 2007; 61(4): 645-652.

[9] Lloyd K M, Dennis M. Cowden's disease. A possible new symptom complex with multiple system involvement. *Ann. Intern. Med.* 1963; 58: 136-142.

[10] Pilarski R, Burt R, Kohlman W, et al. Cowden syndrome and the PTEN hamartoma tumor syndrome: systematic review and revised diagnostic criteria. *J. Natl. Cancer Inst.* 2013; 105(21): 1607-1616.

[11] Wade T R, Kopf A W. Cowden's disease; a case report and review of the literature. *J. Dermatol. Surg. Oncol.* 1978; 4(56): 459-464.

[12] Myers M P, Stolarov J P, Eng C, et al. P-TEN, the tumor suppressor from human chromosome 10q23, is a dual-specificity phosphatase. *Proc. Natl. Acad. Sci. U S A.* 1997; 94(17):9052–9057.

[13] Squarize C H, Castilho R M, Gutkind JS. Chemoprevention and treatment of experimental Cowden's disease by mTOR inhibition with rapamycin. *Cancer Res.* 2008;68(17):7066–7072.

[14] Tashiro H, Blazes M S, Wu R, et al. Mutations in PTEN are frequent in endometrial carcinoma but rare in other common gynecological malignancies. *Cancer Res.* 1997; 57(18):3935–3940.

[15] Kurose K, Gilley K, Matsumoto S, et al. Frequent somatic mutations in PTEN and TP53 are mutually exclusive in the stroma of breast carcinomas. *Nat. Genet.* 2002; 32(3):355–357.

[16] Gast A, Scherer D, Chen B, et al. Somatic alterations in the melanoma genome: a high-resolution array-based comparative genomic hybridization study. *Genes Chromosomes Cancer.* 2010;49(8):733–745.

[17] Gammon A, Jasperson K, Champine M. Genetic basis of Cowden syndrome and its implications for clinical practice and risk management. *Appl. Clin. Genet.* 2016; 9: 83-92.

[18] Ni Y, Zbuk K M, Sadler T, et al. Germline mutations and variants in the succinate dehydrogenase genes in Cowden and Cowden-like syndromes. *Am. J. Hum. Genet.* 2008; 83(2): 261-268.

[19] Ni Y, He X, Chen J, et al. Germline SDHx variants modify breast and thyroid cancer risks in Cowden and Cowden-like syndrome via FAD/NAD-dependent destabilization of p53. *Hum. Mol. Genet.* 2012; 21(2): 300-310.

[20] Bennett K L, Mester J, Eng C. Germline epigenetic regulation of KILLIN in Cowden and Cowden-like syndrome. *JAMA* 2010; 304(24): 222-233.

[21] The National Comprehensive Cancer Network (NCCN). The NCCN guidelines genetic/familial high-risk assessment: Breast and ovarian. *J. Natl. Compr. Cancer Netw.* 2017; 15: 9-20.

[22] Abel T W, Baker S J, Fraser M M, et al. Lhermitte-Duclos disease: a report of 31 cases with immunohistochemical analysis of the PTEN/AKT/mTOR pathway. *J. Neuropathol. Exp. Neurol.* 2005; 64(4): 341-349.

[23] Albrecht S, Haber R M, Goodman J C, et al. Cowden syndrome and Lhermitte-Duclos disease. *Cancer* 1992; 70(4): 869-876.

[24] Starink T M, van der Veen JP, Arwert F, et al. The Cowden syndrome: a clinical and genetic study in 21 patients. *Clin. Genet.* 1986; 29(3): 222-233.

[25] Nelen M R, Kremer H, Konings I B. et al. Novel PTEN mutations in patients with Cowden disease: absence of clear genotype-phenotype correlations. *Eur. J. Hum. Genet.* 1999; 7(3): 267-273.

[26] Riegert-Johnson D L, Gleeson F C, Roberts M, et al. Cancer and Lhermitte-Duclos disease are common in Cowden syndrome patients. *Hered Cancer Clin. Pract.* 2010; 8(1): 6.

[27] Giorgianni A, Pellegrino C, De Benedictis A, et al. Lhermitte-Duclos disease. A case report. *Neuroradiol. J.* 2013; 26(6): 655-660.

[28] Wei G, Zhang W, Li Q, et al. Magnetic resonance characteristics of adult-onset Lhermitte-Duclos disease: An indicator for active cancer surveillance? *Mol. Clin. Oncol.* 2014; 2(3): 415-420.

[29] Milbouw G, Born J D, Martin D, et al. Clinical and radiological aspects of dysplastic cerebellar gangliocytoma (Lhermitte-Duclos disease); a report of two cases with review of the literature. *Neurosurgery* 1988; 22(1 Pt 1): 124-128.

[30] Thomas B, Krishnamoorthy T, Radhakrishnan W, et al. Advanced MR imaging in Lhermitte-Duclos disease: moving closer to pathology and pathophysiology. *Neuroradiology* 2007; 49(9): 733-738.

[31] Hair L S, Symmans F, Powers J M, et al. Immunohistochemistry and proliferative activity in Lhermitte-Duclos disease. *Acta Neuropathol.* 1992; 84(5): 570-573.

[32] Abel T W, Baker S J, Fraser M M, et al. Lhermitte-Duclos disease: a report of 31 cases with immunohistochemical analysis of the PTEN/AKT/mTOR pathway. *J. Neuropathol. Exp. Neurol.* 2005; 64(4): 341-349.

[33] Schindler G, Capper D, Meyer J, et al. Analysis of BRAF V600E mutation in 1,320 nervous system tumors reveals high mutation frequencies in pleomorphic xanthoastrocytoma, ganglioglioma and extra-cerebellar pilocytic astrocytoma. *Acta Neuropathol.* 2011; 121(3): 397-405.

[34] Williams D W III, Elster A D, Ginsber L E, et al. Recurrent Lhermitte-Duclos diseae: report of two cases and association with Cowden's disease. *AJNR Am. J. Neuroradiol.* 1992; 13: 287-290.

In: Tumors of the Central Nervous System   ISBN: 978-1-53619-628-3
Editor: James A. Reed   © 2021 Nova Science Publishers, Inc.

Chapter 7

CLINICOPATHOLOGIC REVIEW OF CEREBELLAR LIPONEUROCYTOMA

*Richard A. Prayson**, *MD, MEd*
Cleveland Clinic Department of Anatomic Pathology,
Cleveland, OH, US

ABSTRACT

Cerebellar liponeurocytoma is a rare cerebellar tumor which is marked by admixed neurocytic and lipoma-like components. The lesion is thought to arise from cerebellar progenitor cells. Most patients are adults and the tumor shows no gender predilection. Patients typically present with symptoms of headaches, ataxia, gait disturbances, and signs related to increased intracranial pressure. Histologically, the tumor is marked by sheets of uniformly appearing, rounded cells with intermixed lipid-rich cells. Features typically associated with high grade tumors, such as prominent mitotic activity, necrosis and vascular proliferation, are usually absent. The neurocytic cells typically stain with markers of neuronal differentiation including neuron specific enolase, synaptophysin and MAP-2. Ki-67 cell proliferation indices are typically low, generally in the range of 1-3%. TP53 missense mutations have been noted in about 20%

---

* Corresponding Author's E-mail: praysor@ccf.org.

of tumors. Cerebellar liponeurocytomas are considered World Heath Organization (WHO) grade II neoplasms. Most patients have a favorable prognosis, with survival in excess of 5 years. A subset of tumors do recur and recurrent tumors may show evidence of increased mitotic figures, necrosis or vascular proliferation.

This chapter will review the clinicopathologic features of these neoplasms.

INTRODUCTION

Cerebellar lipneurocytoma is a rare tumor that was first described in 1978 by Bechtal and colleagues [1]. They reported a case of a 44-year-old male who presented with an unsteady gait, left facial numbness, slurred speech and an occipital headache. He was noted to have a right cerebellar hemispheric mass. The patient expired 18 hours following a posterior exploratory procedure.

At autopsy, a large hemispheric mass was noted. The lesion was described as showing multiple islets of mature adipose tissue separated and intermixed with a neuroectodermal tumor of mixed components with features of what they described as medulloblastoma and astrocytoma. They designated the lesion as a mixed mesenchymal and neuroectodermal tumor of the cerebellum.

The tumor has historically been referred to by a number of other names including neurolipocytoma, medullocytoma, lipomatous glioneurocytoma, and lipidized mature neuroectodermal tumor of the cerebellum [2-5]. The World Health Organization (WHO) adopted the designation of cerebellar liponeurocytoma in order to emphasize the neurocytomatous nature of the tumor and to distinguish it form medulloblastoma [6, 7].

The tumor currently is recognized as a WHO grade II neoplasm in the most recent version of the WHO classification schema [6]. In its initial inclusion in the WHO schema in 2000, it was designated as a grade I tumor and placed under the general category of a glioneuronal tumor [8]. In the 2007 version of the WHO schema, the tumor's grade was revised to Grade II [9].

CLINICAL FEATURES

The mean age of presentation of cerebellar liponeurocytomas is about 50 years (age range 24-77 years) [6]. There is no definite gender predilection for the tumor [10, 11].

Rare reports of tumors arising in a familial setting have been documented; in one case, this involved two sisters and in the other, a mother and daughter [12, 13].

The majority of tumors arise in the cerebellum, most frequently in the hemispheres, but occasional cases may originate in the vermis or paramedian regions. Rare cases have presented as an exophytic mass extending into the cerebellopontine angle region [14].

Rare reports of these tumors arising in other locations including the lateral and third ventricles and supratentorial region have been documented [15-17]; these have been sometimes referred to as central neuroliponeurocytomas.

The most commonly reported clinical manifestations of these tumors included headaches and symptoms related to increased intracranial pressure.

The later may be directly due to the tumor or due to obstructive hydrocephalus related to the tumor. Some patients present with cerebellar signs including disturbed gait or ataxia.

On imaging studies, cerebellar liponeurocytomas typically present as circumscribed masses. On computed tomography (CT) studies, the tumor may be variably hypodense or isodense with focal regions of hypoattentuation related to the amount of adipose tissue in the tumor [14, 18]. The tumors are heterogeneously enhancing in appearance on T1-weighted magnetic resonance imaging (MRI), with areas of hyperintensity corresponding to the lipid-rich cellular component within the neoplasm. Edema is not usually a salient finding in these tumors, since they are typically slow growing [19].

Enhancement with gadolinium is usually heterogeneous. On T2-weighted MRI studies, the neoplasm is slightly hyperintense. Multifocal tumor has been rarely reported [20].

PATHOLOGY

Histologically, these tumors are marked by an admixture of two elements: a round cell proliferation and intermixed lipomatous component (Figure 1). The adipocyte component can be variably distributed in the tumor and can vary in amount but resembles benign adipose tissue (Figure 2). Interestingly, these cells are not true fat cells but are neuroepithelial tumor cells with increased lipid accumulation in their cytoplasm, causing them to look very much like fat cells. The neurocytic component is comprised of generally rounded cells with clear or lightly eosinophilic cytoplasm and ill-defined cell membranes, resembling the tumor cells seen in central neurocytomas (Figure 3). Neurocytomatous rosettes have been occasionally described. Vascular proliferative changes and necrosis are generally absent in these tumors. Most cases show few if any mitotic figures. Ultrastructural studies have confirmed the neural differentiation of the tumor by highlighting the presence of dense core granules, microtubules and synapse-like structures [4, 21].

Cell proliferation labelling indices are typically low in cerebellar liponeurocytomas. Ki-67 or MIB-1 indices are typically in the 1 - 3% range and may be as high as 6% [2, 22, 23]. The cells with increased lipid appear to be less proliferative in the tumor.

Rare cases of recurrent tumor have been reported and in some of those instances, features typically associated with higher grade lesions such as necrosis, nuclear atypia and vascular proliferation may be evident; the lipidized cellular component in these recurrent tumors also appears to be reduced [4, 24]. A higher Ki-67 labeling index has also been noted in recurrent tumors, as high as 10% in one report [24].

As is the case with other neurocytic tumors of the central nervous system, cerebellar liponeurocytomas also stain with antibodies that target neural-differentiated cells, such as neuron specific enolase, synaptophysin, and MAP-2.

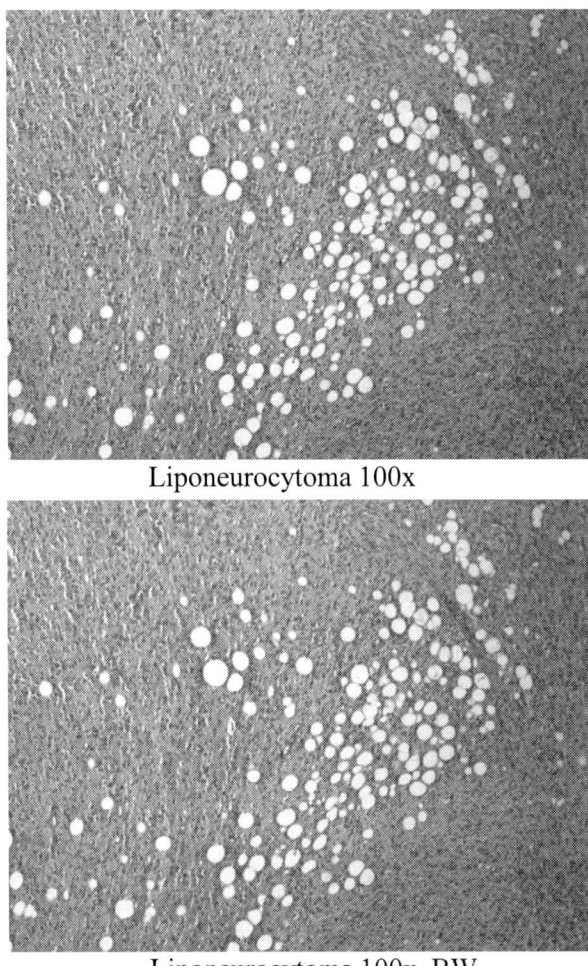

Figure 1. Low magnification appearance of a cerebellar liponeurocytoma showing an admixture of adipocyte cells and small round neurocytic cells (hematoxylin and eosin, original magnification 100X).

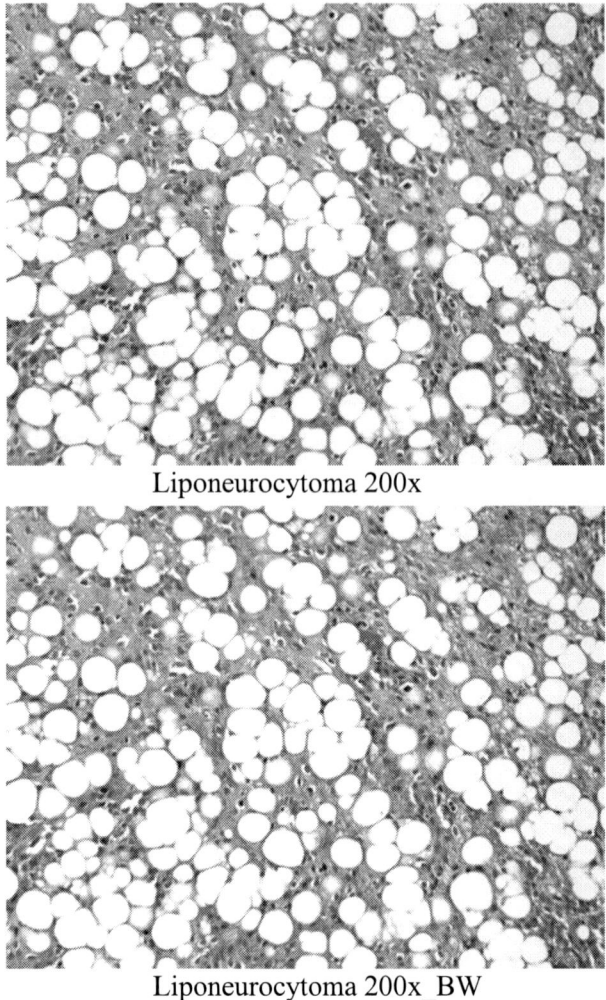

Liponeurocytoma 200x

Liponeurocytoma 200x_BW

Figure 2. An area showing a predominate number of adipocyte cells (hematoxylin and eosin, original magnification 200X).

Tumors may also show focal areas of glial differentiation, as evidenced by glial fibrillary acidic protein immunostaining [3, 23]. A rare tumor has also been documented to show evidence of myoid or ependymal differentiation [5, 25].

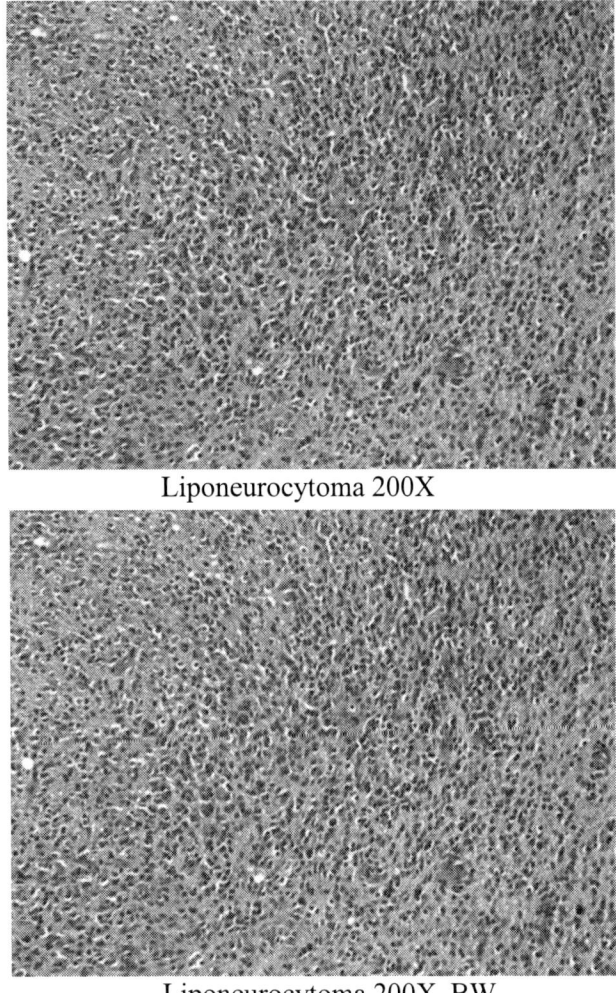

Figure 3. An area resembling an extraventricular neurocytoma, devoid of adipocyte cells (hematoxylin and eosin, original magnification 200X).

GENETIC AND MOLECULAR FEATURES

In one study of 20 cerebellar liponeurocytomas, it was noted that 4 tumors demonstrated evidence of TP53 mutations; abnormalities typically associated with medulloblastomas such as isochromosome 17q, PTCH mutations, CTNNB1 mutations and APC mutations are not features of the cerebellar liponeurocytoma [10]. Gene expression profile analyses of these tumors show features more closely aligned with neurocytomas than medulloblastomas [10]. The TP53 alteration, seen in a minority of cases, is not a finding encountered in medulloblastomas and may indicate tumor development via a different pathway than is seen with neurocytomas. Work done by Anghileri et al. noted that transcription factor NGN1 is expressed in cerebellar liponeurocytomas, a finding not seen in normal adult cerebellar tissue [26].

They also noted that adipocyte fatty-acid-binding protein, which is usually seen in adipocytes, was also overexpressed in the cerebellar liponeurocytoma cells as compared with normal cerebellar tissue. They suggested that the tumor may arise from cerebellar progenitor cells, distinct from cerebellar granule progenitors.

DIFFERENTIAL DIAGNOSIS

The primary differential diagnostic consideration is with medulloblastoma. Medulloblastomas typically arise in pediatric patients and may also demonstrate evidence of neural differentiation by immunostaining.

Morphologically, medulloblastomas typically demonstrate features of high grade tumors including prominent mitotic activity and necrosis. The tumor cells in medulloblastoma often have a more primitive embryonal appearance and more frequently demonstrate features of nuclear atypia and anaplasia. The lipidized cytoplasm of cells in the cerebellar liponeurocytoma is generally not a feature of medulloblastoma.

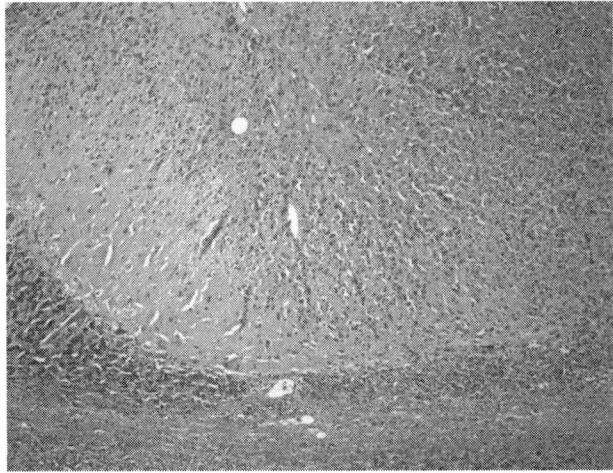
Liponeurocytoma 100x

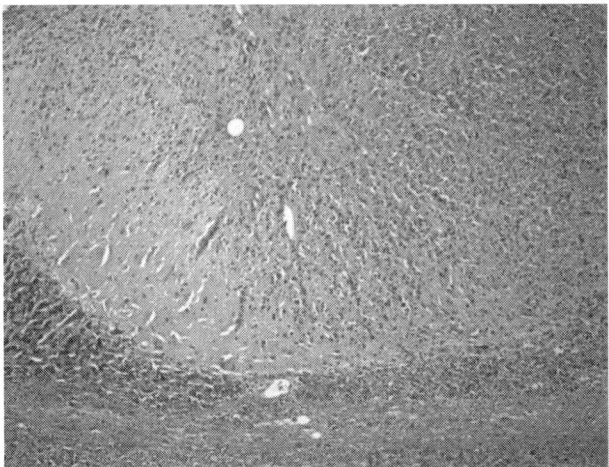
Liponeurocytoma 100x_BW

Figure 4. The liponeurocytoma has an infiltrative border (hematoxylin and eosin, original magnification 100X).

As previously mentioned, the genetic and molecular features of medulloblastomas and cerebellar liponeurocytomas are different.

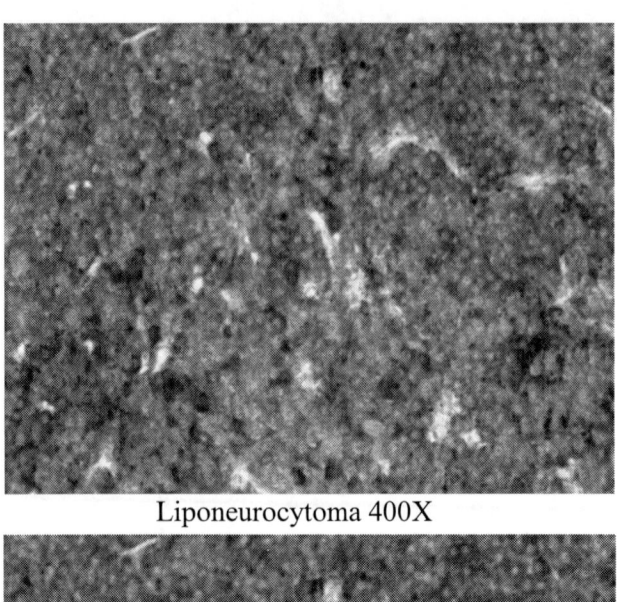
Liponeurocytoma 400X

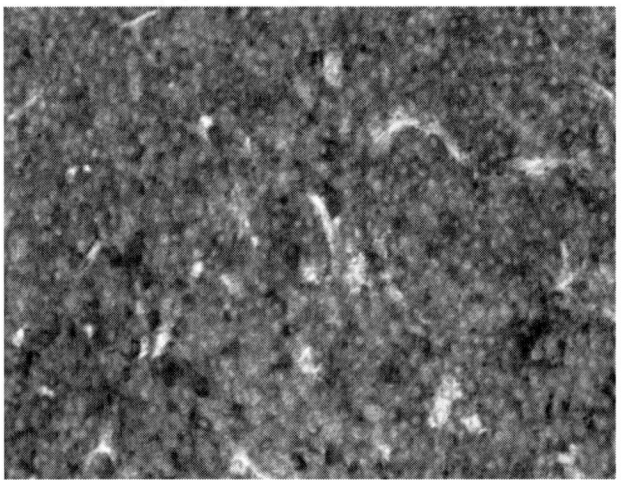
Liponeurocytoma 400X_BW

Figure 5. Diffuse strong synaptophysin immunostaining in a neurocytomatous appearing area of a cerebellar liponeurocytoma (hematoxylin and eosin, original magnification 400X).

TREATMENT AND PROGNOSIS

Although considered low grade neoplasms, a significant number of tumors do recur. In one review, as many as 60% of tumors recurred sometime in up to 12 years of followup [10]. Surgical resection is the treatment of choice. Unfortunately, there are no reliable histologic parameters to predict which tumors are likely to behave in a more aggressive fashion. Radiation may be employed following surgery, particularly in recurrent tumors. The 5 year survival is reported to be 48% with a mean overall survival of 5.8 years [6].

REFERENCES

[1] Bechtel, J. T., Patton, J. M., Takei, Y. Mixed mesenchymal and neuroectodermal tumor of the cerebellum. *Acta Neuropathol.*, (Berl) 1978; 41:261 - 263.

[2] Ellison, D. W., Zygumunt, S. C., Weller, R. O., Neurocytoma/lipoma (neurolipocytoma) of the cerebellum. *Neuropathol. Appl. Neurobiol.*, 1993; 19(1): 95 - 98.

[3] Alleyne, C. H. Jr., Hunter, S., Olson, J. J. et al. Lipomatous glioneurocytoma of the posterior fossa with divergent differentiation: case report. *Neurosurgery,* 1998; 42(3): 639 - 643.

[4] Giangaspero, F., Cennacchi, G., Roncaroli, F. et al. Medullocytoma (lipidized medulloblastoma). A cerebellar neoplasm of adults with favorable prognosis. *Am. J. Surg. Pathol.,* 1996; 20(6): 656 - 664.

[5] Gonzalez-Campora, R., Weller, R. O. Lipidized mature neuroectodermal tumour of the cerebellum with myoid differentiation. *Neuropathol. Appl. Neurobiol.,* 1998; 24(5): 397 - 402.

[6] Kleihues, P., Giangaspero, F., Chimelli, L. et al. Cerebellar liponeurocytoma. In: Louis DN, Ohgaki H, Wiestler OD, et al, Eds) In: *WHO Classification of Tumours of the Central Nervous System.* IARC Press. Lyon, FR. 2016: pp. 161 - 163.

[7] Louis, D. N., Perry, A., Reifenberger, G. et al. The 2016 World Health Organization Classification of Tumors of the Central Nervous System: a summary. *Acta Neuropathol.,* 2016; 131:803 - 820.

[8] Cai, J., Li, W., Du, J. et al. Supratentorial intracerebral cerebellar liponeurocytoma. *Medicine,* 2018; 97(2): e9556.
[9] Louis, D. N., Ohgaki, H., Wiestler, O. D. et al. The 2007 WHO classification of tumours of the central nervous system. *Acta Neuropathol.,* 2007; 114:97 - 109.
[10] Horstmann, S., Perry, A., Reifenberger, G. et al. Genetic and expression profiles of cerebellar liponeurocytomas. *Brain Pathol.,* 2004; 14(3): 281 - 289.
[11] Patel, N., Fallah, A., Provias, J., Jha, N. K. Cerebellar liponeurocytoma. *Can. J. Surg.,* 2009; 52:E117 - 9.
[12] Pikis, S., Fellig, Y., Margolin, E. Cerebellar liponeurocytoma in two siblings suggests a possible familial predisposition. *J. Clin. Neurosci.,* 2016; 32:154 - 156.
[13] Wolf, A., Alghefari, H., Krivosheya, D. et al. Cerebellar liponeurocytoma: a rare intracranial tumor with possible familial predisposition. Case report. *J. Neurosurg.,* 2016; 125:57 - 61.
[14] Nishimoto, T., Kanya, B. Cerebellar liponeurocytoma. *Arch. Pathol. Lab. Med.,* 2012; 136(8): 965 - 969.
[15] George, D., Scheithauer, B. Central liponeurocytoma: case report. *Am. J. Surg. Pathol.,* 2001; 25:1551 - 1555.
[16] Kuchelmeister, K., Nestler, U., Siekmann, R. et al. Liponeurocytoma of the left lateral ventricle--case report and review of the literature. *Clin. Neuropathol.,* 2006; 25:86 - 94.
[17] Gupta, K., Salunke, P., Kalra, I., Vasishta, R. K. Central liponeurocytoma: case report and review of literature. *Clin. Neuropathol.,* 2011; 30:80 - 85.
[18] Alkadhi, H., Keller, M., Brandner, S. et al. Neuroimaging of cerebellar liponeurocytoma. Case report. *J. Neurosurg.,* 2001; 95(2): 324 - 331.
[19] Akhaddar, A., Zrara, I., Gazzaz, M. et al. Cerebellar liponeurocytomas (lipomatous medulloblastoma). *J. Neuroradiol.,* 2003; 30(2): 121 - 126.
[20] Scoppetta, T. L. P., Brito, M. C., Prado, J. L. M. et al. Multifocal cerebellar liponeurocytoma. *Neurology,* 2015; 85(21): 1912.

[21] Fung, K. M., Fang, W., Norton, R. E. et al. Cerebellar central liponeurocytoma. *Ultrastruct. Pathol.,* 2003; 27(2): 109 - 114.

[22] Kachhara, R., Bhattacharya, R. N., Nair, S. et al. Liponeurocytoma of the cerebellum – a case report. *Neurol. India,* 2003; 51(2): 274 - 276.

[23] Soylemezoglu, F., Soffer, D., Onol, B. et al. Lipomatous medulloblastoma in adults. A distinct clinicopathological entity. *Am. J. Surg. Pathol.,* 1996; 20(4): 413 - 418.

[24] Radke, J., Gehlhaar, C., Lenze, D. et al. The evolution of the anaplastic cerebellar liponeurocytoma: case report and review of the literature. *Clin. Neuropathol.,* 2015; 34:19 - 25.

[25] Jouvet, A., Lellouch-Tubiana, A., Boddaert, N. et al. Fourth ventricle neurocytoma with lipomatous and ependymal differentiation: a case report. *Acta Neuropathol.,* 2005; 109:346 - 351.

[26] Anghileri, E., Eoli, M., Paterna, R. et al. FABP4 is a candidate marker of cerebellar liponeurocytoma. *J. Neurooncol.,* 2012; 108(3): 513 - 519.

INDEX

#

1p/19q co-deletion, 23, 25

A

acidic, ix, x, 6, 23, 46, 51, 57, 60, 64, 73, 86
adipocyte, 84, 85, 86, 87, 88
adipocyte fatty-acid-binding protein, 88
adipose tissue, 82, 83, 84
age, 4, 5, 9, 10, 11, 18, 19, 32, 46, 58, 72, 83
aggregation, ix, 45, 48, 73, 74
anaplastic ependymoma, 10, 55
anaplastic ganglioglioma, 25
angiocentric glioma, v, vii, ix, 45, 46, 47, 48, 49, 50, 51, 52, 53, 54, 55, 56
antidiuretic hormone, 63
antigen, 6, 37, 51, 60, 63
APC mutations, 88
astrocytes, 18, 23, 46
astrocytoma, 25, 26, 27, 46, 48, 50, 54, 80, 82
asymptomatic, x, 57

ataxia, xi, 72, 81, 83
atypical teratoid/rhabdoid tumor, 10, 14

B

bacteria, 38
benign, vii, viii, 5, 20, 31, 32, 38, 39, 59, 84
biological behavior, 3
blood, ix, 45, 46, 47, 49, 52, 72, 73, 76
blood flow, 72
blood vessels, ix, 45, 46, 47, 49, 52, 73
BRAF V600E mutation, 23, 37, 42, 52, 75, 80
$BRAF^{V600E}$, 62, 67
brain, vii, viii, 1, 2, 4, 11, 12, 13, 14, 15, 18, 28, 48, 50, 58, 59, 70
brain tumor, 2, 4, 11, 12, 13, 14, 15, 28, 58, 59, 70
brainstem, 19, 47
breast cancer, 71
breast carcinoma, 78

C

C19MC amplification, 8, 9, 10, 11
calcification, 48, 59, 66
CD1a, ix, 32, 33, 37, 38
CD31, 60
CD34, x, 23, 25, 26, 58, 60
CD68, ix, 32, 33, 36, 38
CD99, 6, 51, 58, 65
cell cycle, 70
cell line, 15
cell membranes, 84
central, v, vii, ix, 2, 11, 12, 13, 14, 18, 31, 32, 40, 46, 53, 55, 56, 57, 58, 64, 77, 83, 84, 85, 91, 92, 93
central nervous system, vii, ix, 2, 11, 12, 13, 14, 18, 31, 32, 40, 46, 53, 57, 58, 64, 85, 92
central neuroliponeurocytoma, 83
cerebellar liponeurocytoma, vi, vii, xi, 81, 82, 83, 84, 85, 87, 88, 89, 90, 91, 92, 93
cerebellum, 9, 19, 70, 73, 77, 82, 83, 91, 93
cerebral cortex, viii, 18, 20
cerebral hemisphere, 4
cervical lymphadenopathy, 32
chemotherapy, 26, 29, 39, 43, 53, 64
childhood, 2, 4, 14
children, 13, 28, 32, 46, 58
chordoid gliomas, v, vii, ix, 57, 58, 61, 62, 65
chromogranin, 51, 73
chromosomal abnormalities, 52
chromosome, viii, 1, 2, 9, 23, 52, 77
chromosome 10, 77
chromosome 11p11.2, 52
chromosome 1p/19q co-deletion, 23
CKD4, 60
CKN2A aberration, 60
classification, vii, 1, 2, 3, 4, 9, 12, 14, 22, 53, 58, 64, 70, 82, 92
clinical presentation, 55, 60
clinical symptoms, 33, 72
complex DNET, 22, 25, 26
complications, x, 11, 58, 63, 64
composite/mixed ganglioglioma and DNET, 25
cortex, viii, 18, 20, 21, 25, 48, 51, 70
corticosteroid therapy, 42, 43
Cowden disease, 70, 71, 72, 76, 77, 79
craniopharyngioma, 60, 66
craniopharyngiomas, 60
cytoplasm, x, 20, 22, 34, 57, 60, 62, 63, 84, 88

D

dense core granule, 84
diabetes, 33
diabetes insipidus, 33
diagnostic criteria, 71, 77
DICER1 mutation, viii, 2, 5, 9
DICER1 predisposition syndrome, 5, 9
differential diagnosis, 10, 52
diffuse astrocytoma, 48, 50, 53
dysembryoplastic neuroepithelial tumor, v, vii, viii, 17, 18, 27, 28, 29
dysmorphic neurons, 48
dysplasia, viii, ix, 18, 21, 23, 26, 45, 48, 51, 54, 55
dysplastic cerebellar gangliocytoma, vii, x, 69, 70, 72, 73, 74, 75, 76, 77, 79

E

edema, 4, 20, 24, 37, 60
EGFR, 60
embryonal tumor, v, vii, viii, 1, 2, 3, 4, 5, 6, 7, 8, 9, 10, 11, 12, 13, 14, 15
embryonal tumor with abundant neuropil and true rosettes, viii, 1, 2, 8, 12
embryonal tumor with multilayered rosettes, 2, 13, 14, 15

embryonic stem cells, 8
emperipolesis, ix, 32, 33, 38
endometrial carcinoma, 71, 78
eosinophilic granular bodies, 24, 53, 74
ependymal, x, 3, 10, 51, 58, 65, 86, 93
ependymal cell, x, 58
ependymoblastic rosette, 3, 10, 12
ependymoblastoma, viii, 1, 2, 3, 5, 10, 12
ependymoma, 3, 10, 46, 48, 52, 54, 55
epidermoid cyst, 58, 65
epilepsy, ix, 19, 26, 28, 29, 45, 46, 47, 48, 54, 55
epithelial, 6, 37, 51, 60, 63, 71
epithelial growth factor, 60
epithelial membrane antigen, 6, 37, 51, 60, 63
Epstein-Barr virus, 39
Erdheim-Chester disease, 37, 42
evidence, viii, ix, x, xi, 1, 3, 8, 45, 52, 55, 69, 75, 82, 86, 87, 88

F

facial nerve, 47
factor 1, x, 58, 60, 67
FGFR1 mutation, 25
focal cortical dysplasia, viii, ix, 18, 21, 23, 26, 45, 48, 51, 55
focal seizure, viii, 17, 24

G

ganglioglioma, viii, x, 18, 19, 25, 26, 69, 73, 75, 80
ganglion, x, 5, 70, 73
ganglion cells, x, 5, 70, 73
ganglioneuroma, 76
gene expression, 7
generalized tonic-clonic seizure, 19
glial fibrillary acidic protein (GFAP), ix, x, 6, 10, 23, 46, 51, 58, 60, 64, 73, 86

glioma, x, 3, 24, 25, 46, 48, 49, 50, 51, 52, 53, 54, 55, 56, 57, 58, 61, 63, 64, 65, 66, 67, 68, 69, 73
growth, 7, 10, 46, 47, 50, 60, 73

H

histiocytes, ix, 32, 33, 34, 35, 36, 38
Homer-Wright, 9
human herpesvirus type 6, 39
hybridization, 52, 60, 78
hydrocephalus, x, 69, 72, 83
hypermethylation, 71
hypertrophy, 70, 76
hypopituitarism, 33
hypothalamic dysfunction, 59, 63
hypothalamus, 63
hypothesis, 58

I

IgG4, 37, 38, 42, 43
images, 20, 47, 59
imbalances, 60
immune system, 39
immunoglobulin, 39
immunohistochemistry, 33, 37
immunomarkers, x, 51, 70
immunoreactivity, 14, 36, 37
in situ hybridization, 3, 39, 62
interface, 47, 48, 50, 74
intracranial pressure, x, xi, 4, 69, 72, 81, 83
isochromosome 17q, 87
Isocitrate dehydrogenase (IDH)- 1 and -2 mutations, 23

K

Ki-67, xi, 23, 51, 60, 73, 81, 84
KRAS, 39, 44

L

Langerhans cell histiocytosis, 37, 41
lesions, ix, x, 31, 32, 33, 37, 45, 52, 69, 70, 71, 72, 73, 76, 84
Lhermitte-Duclos disease, vi, vii, x, 69, 70, 71, 73, 77, 78, 79
lipoma, vii, xi, 81, 91
liponeurocytomas, xi, 82, 83, 84, 85, 87, 89, 92
lymph, 32, 33, 39, 40, 41, 43
lymphadenopathy, 32, 33, 39, 40, 41, 43
lymphocytes, 33, 34, 61

M

macrocephaly, 71, 72
magnetic resonance imaging, x, 47, 57, 59, 83
MAP2K1 mutation, 39, 44
MDM2 amplifications, 60
medulloblastoma, 2, 9, 82, 88, 91, 92, 93
medulloepithelioma, viii, 1, 3, 5, 8, 9, 12, 13
membrane antigen, 6, 51, 60, 63
meningioma, 33, 37, 40, 41, 58, 60, 62, 64
meningiomas, ix, 31, 33, 37, 41, 59, 63
mutations, viii, x, xi, 2, 9, 23, 25, 29, 39, 41, 42, 43, 44, 52, 56, 62, 69, 70, 71, 75, 76, 78, 79, 81, 87
myelin-oligodendrocyte glycoprotein, 23

N

necrosis, ix, x, xi, 25, 45, 53, 59, 60, 69, 73, 81, 84, 88
neoplasm, vii, viii, ix, x, 17, 18, 46, 49, 54, 57, 67, 70, 82, 83, 84, 91
neuroblastic, 9, 12
neurocytomatous rosette, 84
neuroectodermal tumors, viii, 1, 2
neurofibromatosis type 1, 19, 28
neurofilament, 6, 73
neurofilament protein, 6
neuroimaging, 13, 37, 66
neuroliponeurocytomas, 83
neurologic symptom, 38
neuron specific enolase, xi, 23, 81, 85
neuronal cells, x, 20, 25, 26, 27, 70, 73
neurons, viii, 18, 20, 22, 23, 24, 48, 51, 73
NGN1, 88
non-specific DNET, 22
nuclei, 5, 10, 22, 24, 34, 38, 48, 60, 62, 75

O

obstructive, x, 69, 72, 83
obstructive hydrocephalus, x, 69, 72, 83
olig2, 23
oligodendrocytes, 18
oligodendroglia, 20
oligodendroglioma, viii, 18, 24, 25, 27, 28

P

pharmacoresistent epilepsy, ix, 45, 47
pilocytic astrocytoma, 53, 80
pilomyxoid astrocytoma, 53
plasma cells, 33, 34, 38, 43, 61
primitive, viii, 1, 2, 3, 5, 6, 7, 9, 10, 12, 13, 14, 88
primitive neuroectodermal tumor, viii, 1, 2, 12, 13
PRKCA gene, 62
progenitor cell, xi, 81, 88
progesterone, 37, 63
progesterone receptor, 37, 63
prognosis, viii, ix, xi, 2, 11, 26, 46, 59, 82, 91
proliferation, ix, x, xi, 22, 23, 25, 45, 47, 51, 53, 55, 57, 60, 71, 73, 81, 84
pseudorosettes, 9, 46, 48

psychotic symptoms, 47, 54
PTCH, 87
PTCH mutations, 88
pulmonary embolism, 63

R

radiation, 11, 13, 26, 29, 38, 53, 91
radiation therapy, 39, 53
recurrence, x, 26, 38, 52, 55, 59, 63, 64, 70, 76
related disease, 37, 38, 39, 42, 43
renal cell carcinoma, 71
resection, x, 11, 26, 38, 58, 63, 70, 76, 91
Rosai-Dorfman disease, v, vii, viii, 31, 32, 34, 35, 36, 39, 40, 41, 42, 43, 44, 58

S

S-100 protein, ix, 33, 36, 37, 38, 46, 51, 60
secondary, 53
seizures, viii, 4, 17, 18, 19, 24, 26, 27, 46, 63, 72
simple DNET, 19, 20, 26
sinus histiocytosis with massive lymphadenopathy, 32, 39, 40, 41, 43
somatic mutations, 71, 78
somatostatin receptor 2a, 37, 63
somatostatin receptor 2a (SSTR2a), 37, 63
structures of Sherer, 53
subarachnoid hemorrhage, 72
surgical intervention, 38, 47
surgical resection, ix, 26, 38, 46, 53, 63, 76
survival, xi, 8, 11, 26, 55, 63, 64, 71, 82, 91
symptoms, x, xi, 4, 19, 33, 47, 57, 59, 69, 72, 81, 83

synaptophysin, x, xi, 6, 8, 10, 23, 51, 60, 62, 70, 73, 81, 85, 90
syndrome, x, 5, 9, 40, 43, 63, 69, 71, 77, 78, 79
syndrome of inappropriate antidiuretic hormone, 63

T

temporal lobe, vii, viii, 17, 19, 24, 47, 55
temporal lobe epilepsy, 55
therapy, viii, 2, 13
thyroid, x, 5, 58, 60, 67, 70, 71, 78
thyroid transcription, x, 58, 60, 67
thyroid transcription factor 1, x, 58, 60, 67
tissue, viii, 8, 18, 38, 73, 76, 88
Touton-type multinucleated giant cells., 38
true rosettes, viii, 1, 2, 5, 8, 10, 12, 52
tumor cells, 7, 9, 37, 48, 49, 53, 60, 62, 84, 88
tumor development, 88
tumorigenesis, 71

V

ventricle, ix, 47, 57, 59, 65, 66, 67, 68, 92, 93
vessels, 3, 33, 47, 53
visual acuity, 59
vomiting, 4, 33, 59

X

XYY syndrome, 19, 28